TABLE OF CONTENTS

PART 1:
OVERVIEW

INTRODUCTION

Ever since I was a youth athlete, I've endeavored to improve my health and athletic performance. My interest in health and fitness grew as I read dozens of health books and became a World Instructor Training Schools-certified personal fitness trainer and a National Academy of Sports Medicine-certified fitness nutrition specialist and youth fitness trainer. Through a combination of reading fitness books, completing certifications, and putting theory to practice in the real world, I've come to love using sandbag training in my workouts.

Old-school sandbag training isn't as flashy as newfangled fitness trends like vibration plates and balance boards, but its no-frills essence is precisely why sandbag training is so effective. Fancy, complicated training methods can sound appealing at first, but simplicity is a strength, not a weakness. The simpler the exercise modality, the fewer barriers there are to a good workout. When training with a sandbag, the only thing you need to think about is the single bag in front of you. You're essentially just picking up, pressing, and carrying large, awkward objects—a perfect training method that prepares you for everyday activities like moving furniture, carrying groceries, and going on backpacking trips.

So let it be known, sandbag training is not some passing fad. Whether you're a desk jockey or a professional athlete, incorporating sandbag training into your fitness regimen will take standard bodyweight moves to a whole new level.

WHY SANDBAG TRAINING?

Training with a sandbag isn't easy, and that's the point. If your workout allows you to idly chat with a friend without breaking a sweat, it probably isn't making you stronger. Don't get it twisted—your workout doesn't need to kill you in order for it to be effective. But it does have to give your body a challenge, and using sandbags—essentially resistance training—is a great way to do that.

Incorporating sandbags in resistance training is great for both men and women. When done properly, it's helpful for nearly all fitness goals, including fat loss, muscle gain, health improvement, and athletic development. This is because resistance training excels at one of the most important facets of any exercise modality: muscle engagement. Aerobic training methods like running, jumping rope, and biking are all awesome, healthy things to do. However, aerobic activities don't work the musculature as effectively or efficiently as straight-up resistance training, making resistance training an unparalleled way to develop a fit-looking, strong body.

The biggest advantage to using a sandbag is its large, awkward, unstable nature. This forces your body to recruit the oft-neglected stabilizer muscles and engage in the movement from head to toe. Training in this ultra-functional manner means more metabolic benefits and a stronger body. Sandbag training aims to combine the benefits of intentional, high-load barbell training and real-world manual labor.

Sandbags are also relatively inexpensive and portable. If you buy or make one, your house becomes your gym—no membership fees, commute, or interminable wait for equipment to become available. And when compared to the cost of a full home gym, sandbags are incredibly cost-effective, portable, and take up very little storage space.

Adaptability is another benefit of sandbag training. Many personal trainers have a single training philosophy. Some are proponents of heavy resistance training, others prefer calisthenic circuits, and others are adamant endurance advocates. Sandbags can be incorporated into all those methods, allowing you total flexibility to switch between different training goals.

TRAINING SMART

Personally, I believe there's no one, universal best way for everyone to train because all of us have different preferences and goals. My general training philosophy is constructed from ten primary workout principles. They're as follows:

1. TRAIN WITH FUNCTIONAL, COMPOUND MOVEMENTS. Working small muscles through small ranges of motion makes no sense. Exercising in that way provides a much smaller metabolic benefit and a smaller hormonal response. Additionally, big, multi-joint movements build functional strength, which is beneficial for sports and daily life. Functional, compound exercises make sense because they're much more efficient and effective at helping you hit your workout goals.

2. TRAIN THE WHOLE BODY. Neglecting certain muscle groups or movement patterns can lead to muscle imbalances, which are bad on both a functional and aesthetic level. Besides looking funny, muscle imbalances can affect our posture and movement patterns, and sometimes even lead to injury. To avoid this trap, train your whole body from head to toe!

3. PUT IN AT LEAST A GOOD EFFORT WHEN TRAINING. Unfortunately for the throngs of people who go to the gym to slowly walk on a treadmill or pedal on an exercise bike, half-heartedly exercising isn't particularly helpful for any fitness goals. The body needs to be challenged for exercise to have its full range of positive effects, so be sure to give a good effort at the very least.

4. DON'T FEEL COMPELLED TO DO LONG OR EXTREMELY ARDUOUS WORKOUTS EVERY SINGLE TIME. It isn't necessary to go balls to the wall for every workout to benefit from training. If you're someone with a very high drive, then more power to you. Especially if you're a competitive athlete, you'll get increasing levels of returns from a higher effort. However, long or excruciatingly difficult workouts aren't required for good results. Don't feel like you have to push yourself to the point of sickness for a workout to be worth it. You'll still get immense benefit from working out even if you don't feel 100% spent at the end.

5. DON'T FALL PREY TO ANALYSIS PARALYSIS. Us health nerds love to get bogged down in minutia, and unfortunately the trend has found its way into mainstream health circles. People want their workout to be completely optimal, so they'll spend a lot of time researching and researching until their workout plan is absolutely perfect. Until they read a new article, book, or study, that is. Don't worry about the minutia. A difficult, full-body sandbag workout is going to get you 99% of the benefits that anything else would, so embrace the peace of mind that comes with having a set plan.

6. TRAIN FOR ENJOYMENT, NOT PAIN. One reason people in the developed world don't exercise regularly is that there's a misconception that working out should be painful. This couldn't be farther from the truth. Working out should be made as fun as possible. Why? Because an enjoyable workout will more likely be completed on a consistent basis, and consistency is key for any type of exercise success. Plus, life's too short for self-induced torture. So know thyself and construct an exercise regimen accordingly.

7. CHANGE UP YOUR WORKOUTS CONSTANTLY. Doing the same workout all the time is not only boring, it also produces sub-par results. If we train using the same, exact exercises for long periods of time, our body is able to adapt and we no longer have as much opportunity for growth. So every so often subtract or add some exercises to your regimen to avoid stale workouts.

8. WORK TOWARD A GOAL. Training without a goal makes it impossible to create a proper workout plan, and sharply decreases adherence. Why would you stick to something that doesn't have a clear reason for being in your life? And how do you create a regimen if you don't have an end goal? Even if the goal of your workouts is to have fun, that's a clear directive that can be used to form a workout plan.

9. CUSTOMIZE YOUR WORKOUTS. There's no one-size-fits-all training regimen. A workout plan for a cross-country runner versus one for someone hoping to put on a lot of muscle will look different. Due to our differing genetics, abilities, and, most importantly, our aspirations, we need customized workout plans.

10. ADOPT AN OVERALL HEALTHY LIFESTYLE. Don't make the mistake of using the fact that you work out as an excuse to lead an otherwise unhealthy lifestyle. Working out is wonderful, but it's just one dimension of maintaining overall well-being: Proper sleep, proper nutrition, and avoiding chronic stressors are all crucial if we're to live a long, healthy life.

With these ten training principles in mind, I've included five different training methods to best fit your goals: 1) set and rep training, 2) eustress training, 3) HIT (high-intensity training), 4) circuit training, and 5) endurance training. I detail these methodologies starting on page 17. I also include a number of sample workouts you can either use verbatim or tweak to better fit your goals. Additionally, there are nearly 100 effective exercises detailed with full instructions in Part 3; you can pick and choose from them if you want to construct your own regimens from scratch.

Whether you want to change your body, improve your health, or get an edge on the competition, sandbag training is a fun and effective way to go after your goals.

KEY TERMS & IDEAS

The following are some terms I'll use throughout the book.

TRAINING GOAL: This is what you're working toward when you exercise. Having a goal is important because it helps you decide how you want to construct your workout regimen. A training goal also gives you reason to make time for and put effort into your workouts.

ATHLETIC PERFORMANCE: Athletic performance is a training goal for most athletes. What this means is that when you're striving for this goal, you're focused on improving metrics closely related to your sport rather than working out to be healthy or look a certain way.

BODY COMPOSITION: If you're concerned about how you look, your training goal is body composition. Fat loss is the most common goal because it allows muscle definition to show. Muscle gain is also a common body composition goal as it increases muscle definition as well.

BODYWEIGHT VERSUS BODY FAT: Most people mistakenly talk about losing weight when what they really want to do is lose fat. Losing weight sounds good at first, until you realize that losing weight can also mean losing valuable muscle mass. Muscle tissue is important for both practical and aesthetic reasons. Because of this, judging your results by what your scale says isn't a good idea. In fact, it isn't uncommon at all to gain a pound or two and see a trimmer figure in the mirror. The reason? Muscle weighs more than fat. The solution for those that like to measure their progress is to measure body-fat percentage, which can tell you how much fat you've lost or muscle you've gained when combined with a weight measurement.

OVERTRAINING: Overtraining results from a lack of recovery after workouts. Most people never have to worry about this, but it certainly does happen. Getting sick more often than usual and feeling constantly fatigued and tired are common side effects. To avoid overtraining, be sure to listen to your body and rest when you feel beaten down.

UNDERTRAINING: Undertraining, or not putting in enough effort during your workouts, is much more common than overtraining but doesn't have much in the way of health implications. Undertraining doesn't hamper the immune system, but it does prevent you from getting optimal results.

FREQUENCY: Frequency refers to the number of workouts planned or performed in a certain time period. A high workout frequency would be exercising every day; a low workout frequency would be working out once every week.

INTENSITY: Intensity refers to the difficulty of the workout performed. Intensity is a fairly subjective term as workouts that are intense for some may not be intense for others.

CONSISTENCY: Consistency refers to how often you keep to your workout plans. The more workouts you miss, the less results you'll get from the days you do work out. Be as consistent as possible—consistency is the number-one driver of success.

POSTURE: Posture is the alignment of a body's muscles, bones, and joints. Although modern technologies like computers and cars have been very helpful in many respects, they haven't been good to our collective posture. Specifically, they've caused many people in developed countries to adopt a posture with an overly forward head and neck and a tucked pelvis. Posture can be improved by strengthening the posterior chain and core as well as consciously keeping a high chest and a properly tilted pelvis.

FORM: The form you use while exercising is extremely important in both engaging the proper muscles and avoiding injury. If a particular exercise is giving you trouble, look up a YouTube video to help. It's natural for some movements to be difficult at first; they'll get easier the more you do them. Using your phone camera to take a video of you doing the movement is also a good way to fix any form problems you may have.

POSTERIOR CHAIN: The posterior chain refers to the musculature running across the back of your body. This is the muscle group largely responsible for picking things up off the ground and proper posture. Unfortunately, our modern society has a widespread weakness in the posterior chain muscles. Strengthening the posterior chain should be a big priority for everyone who cares about being strong and pain-free.

CORE: Many people think of the core as simply the abdominal muscles, but the core is actually composed of the muscles around the center of our body. This includes some muscles in the posterior chain, such as our lower back and glutes. A strong core is also very important for being strong and pain-free.

WHOLE-BODY EXERCISE: Like our professional jobs, our workouts have gotten more and more specialized in the modern age. We now have machines that isolate each of our muscles, and fewer of us perform exercises that engage our muscles from head to toe. Although using machines to work each muscle individually may reduce injury-risk in the short run, doing whole-body exercises allows our bodies to use the muscle groups as one.

FUNCTIONAL EXERCISE: A functional exercise is one that translates well to everyday life. A deadlift, for example, is very functional because it simulates lifting something heavy off of the ground. A leg curl machine is not functional as we don't do anything outside of a gym that requires that motion.

UPPER-BODY PUSH: An upper-body push movement is one that requires us to push weight away from our body. A classic example is the chest press (page 37).

UPPER-BODY PULL: An upper-body pull movement is one that requires us to pull weight toward our body. A classic example is the bent-over row.

LOWER-BODY PUSH: A lower-body push movement is one that requires us to push weight away from our body with our legs. A classic example is the squat.

LOWER-BODY PULL: A lower-body pull movement is one that requires us to pull weight with our legs. A classic example is the deadlift.

WARM-UP: This is a set of exercises that prepares the body for training rather than being for the training itself. A warm-up increases performance and decreases chance of injury.

POTENTIAL FOR INJURY: The potential for injury is the risk of injury from a certain movement or workout; the goal is to minimize this. You can do so by always warming up. Another very important way to reduce potential for injury is to listen to your body and understand when you're at your limit. A very common cause of injury is pushing past pain or fatigue, so learning your body's signals is a must.

BEFORE YOU BEGIN

Although working out is a very healthy endeavor, it can be dangerous for a minority of people with certain health risk factors. Do check with a doctor before starting any type of workout regimen.

You'll also want to listen to your body before blindly following a planned workout—if your hamstrings are feeling tight and bothered, going through with your sprint routines may not be the best idea. Adjust your workouts accordingly to reduce the risk of injury. Listening to your body can also help with exercise form, such as if you feel sore in places you shouldn't. On days when your body is feeling great, you can really push it and go for that personal record. On days when you're feeling stiff and vulnerable, training with care may be the best thing to do.

WARMING UP

Warming up is critical if you want to decrease your chance of injury and improve your performance. Training hard with cold muscles straight out of the gate is never a good idea! Starting on page 122, I've recommended a few exercises that are great for warming up. Although many people also advocate doing cool-down exercises after exercising, research has found just a few minutes of walking is really all you need.

A proper warm-up should include some dynamic stretches, which activate your muscles, increase mobility, decrease chance of injury, and improve performance. Static stretching, the kind most of us grew up with, should be avoided pre-exercise as it has been shown to decrease exercise performance in addition to being ineffective at decreasing injury rates.

EQUIPMENT

There are only two vital pieces of equipment needed: a sandbag and a backpack. High-quality sandbags can be found online from a variety of companies. The backpack is needed for weighted exercises where holding a sandbag is either awkward or impossible.

If your sandbags are not durable enough, an optional piece of equipment is a medicine ball, which can be substituted in the throwing exercises.

For those looking to save money or execute a fun DIY project, you can also make your own sandbag:

STEP 1: Fill several gallon-sized zip-top plastic bags halfway full with sand. For sturdier, heavier weights, you can also use heavy-duty ten-gallon zip-top plastic bags.

STEP 2: Reinforce the plastic bags by taping over the entire bag with one layer of heavy-duty tape.

STEP 3: Fill a duffel bag or backpack with the reinforced sandbags.

COMMITMENT TO SUCCESS

For you to successfully integrate exercise into your life, you'll need to have a concrete reason for sticking to your regimen. Exercising *without* a purpose is the best way to sleepwalk through a workout and drop exercising altogether. So be clear on why you're working out. Are you working out for health reasons? To look good in a swimsuit? To improve your performance on the basketball court? To get stronger for everyday life? To have fun and let off steam? Whatever the reason, let it guide your workouts and exercise programming. For detailed information on which kinds of workout regimens are best for specific workout goals, see "Training Methods" on page 17.

With that said, any training routine is worthless if you don't stick with your exercise plan. The best ways to adhere to your regimen are:

1. MAKE SURE YOU ENJOY YOUR WORKOUTS. On a busy day, you're way more likely to get a fun workout in than one that you dread.

2. MAKE SURE YOUR WORKOUTS AREN'T TOO LONG OR ARDUOUS. Yes, pushing yourself physically is fantastic. However, if your workout is so long or difficult that you avoid it, it won't do any good. Start small, and as you consistently make your workouts several months in a row, you can increase the length and difficulty.

3. SCHEDULE YOUR WORKOUTS IN YOUR CALENDAR OR PLANNER AND TREAT THEM LIKE AN IMPORTANT MEETING. Make working out feel as routine as brushing your teeth. If you categorize working out as optional, based on your motivation level that day, your workout attendance will be shaky. But if you schedule your workouts and get used to getting them in no matter what, they'll become instilled as a cornerstone of your habitual life.

HOW TO USE THIS BOOK

Benjamin Franklin once said, "By failing to prepare, you are preparing to fail." Though Mr. Franklin was known more for his intellect rather than his physicality, the world of fitness is a perfect fit for his quote. The first thing many people do upon purchasing a new exercise book is flip around the pages and then immediately jump into the moves that appeal to them. Though enthusiasm is great, jumping right into things without concern for planning, scheduling, and exercise form is not a recipe for sustainable results. This section provides an overview on how to get the most out of this book and maximize your ability to meet your fitness goals.

1. Find your "why."

The first step in creating your sandbag workout routine is identifying why you want to work out in the first place. Create a list of your motivations for exercising, and then circle the one or two that resonate with you the strongest.

2. Pick your training modality and create a workout plan.

Based on your top one or two training goals, pick a workout modality from Part 2. Don't choose a modality based solely on your goals, though; you should also take personal factors into account. For example, if you're the type of person who tends to get impatient with slower, methodical workouts, don't choose eustress training.

Once you've chosen a modality, create your training plan from the sample workouts that are provided in Part 2. Pick the workouts that seem most appealing to you. If you don't end up enjoying them, you can always swap them for another workout. Also, consider starting out with the "essentialist" workouts, which are optimally formulated for each of the common workout goals.

3. Schedule your workouts.

Pick the days you'd like to work out and set reminders on your phone, calendar, or anywhere else that will help you remember your schedule. If you're the type of person who functions best without planning, you can try to commit to an unplanned regimen, but the majority of people do best with a schedule. I'd recommend starting out with a less-intense regimen and then adding in more workouts per week once you've been consistent with your first schedule.

4. Focus on form.

Once your training plan and workout schedule are set, make sure your form is solid before using a heavy sandbag. Use the instructions and pictures in Part 3 as a starting point. Searching the exercise name on YouTube is also a great way to improve your form. The best method of all, however, is to use your smartphone or a video camera to film yourself while performing the exercise, and then tweaking your form based on the footage. Exercising with improper form increases your chance of injury so it's worth the time and effort to get it right.

5. Adjust as you go.

I like to think of my various endeavors as $n=1$ science experiments, and working out is no different. Be tuned in to your workouts so you can figure out what works and what doesn't, what you like and what you don't, and anything else that could help improve your future workouts. After you've run your beta experiment for a month or two, assess your workout plan and make any changes that you feel would be beneficial. Add exercises to workouts, subtract exercises from workouts, or experiment with a different training modality altogether. Your exercise plan is never set in stone, so if something isn't working then make a change.

PART 2:
PROGRAMS

CREATING A CUSTOMIZED WORKOUT

As stated in the previous section, you should have one or more specific reasons why you work out. There are hundreds of valid workout motivations, and your training plan should vary along with your training goals. A mom training for a marathon should be training differently than the grandpa looking to put on muscle. No one workout plan or modality is best suited for every training goal.

The six most common fitness goals I see are fat loss, muscle gain, strength gain, improved athletic performance, improved general health, and improved general conditioning. Oftentimes, people have a combination of these goals. To achieve them, this book details five different training methods, each of which has its own set of pros and cons. These methods are set-and-reps training, eustress training, endurance training, high-intensity training, and circuit training. The following section walks you through these training goals and methods.

FITNESS GOALS

If your fitness goal is *fat loss*, you're looking to drop your body-fat percentage without losing lean muscle mass. The best way to achieve this goal is to focus on healthy eating and follow a training plan that's composed of intense resistance-training routines.

A goal of *muscle gain* means your aim is to add muscle to your frame. You'll want to eat a lot of energy-dense food and employ a workout plan that focuses on lifting heavy weight with enough rest time for your body to recover.

When you want to *gain strength*, your goal is to increase your power output. To accomplish this, your workouts should be centered around consistently lifting heavy weights without switching up your routine too frequently.

Increased athletic performance means improving the strength and coordination of basic movements that transfer to nearly every sport. This will mean workouts with a wide variety of functional movements.

Those looking to improve *general health* want to reduce disease risk factors and improve overall quality of life. The best way to do that is by moving around consistently and challenging your muscles with intense workouts.

General conditioning means keeping your body prepared for whatever fun adventure life throws your way. This can be done by shoring up your weaknesses and embracing a variety of different workouts.

TRAINING METHODS

SETS & REPS TRAINING: The sets and reps method of training is the most common workout plan. Being common isn't a bad thing, however; the popularity of the sets and reps regimen is a testament to its effectiveness. This method is quite versatile and is a great regimen for almost every goal.

A sets and reps workout is performed by doing a set number of repetitions and sets. If you were performing squats, for example, and your regimen called for five sets of five reps, you'd perform five squats, rest for a minute or two, and then perform five reps of squats four more times to complete your five sets of five reps each.

Of course, you might not always hit your target number of sets and reps, which is completely fine. Other times you might be able to exceed your target number of sets and reps, which is also not a problem. The number of sets and reps you set as your target is only what you're shooting for. At the end of the day, what matters is that you're giving your muscles the work they need to get stronger.

Best for: fat loss, muscle gain, increased athletic performance, strength gain, general health

EUSTRESS TRAINING: Eustress training is the least common method I've included in this book, but I think it's poised to increase in popularity in the coming years. This fairly versatile (if a bit unorthodox) training method is best for athletes trying to increase their top-end performance (whether it's sprint speed, jump height, or deadlift weight) or for people who don't like feeling completely wasted and useless after a hard workout.

Eustress workouts are essentially executed by performing many one-rep sets. If you were performing deadlifts, for example, and your regimen called for 50 sets of one rep, you'd perform one deadlift, rest for about 30 seconds, and repeat the deadlift 49 more times to complete your 50 sets of one rep each. Since the goal is to prevent yourself from getting so fatigued that your performance suffers, the rest time is highly variable. Simply rest as long as needed to stay fresh. At first this may be only a few seconds, but by the end of the workout you may require a minute in between reps.

Again, don't get hung up on hitting a certain amount of repetitions. The goal is to increase your strength and practice your form using heavy loads. Accomplishing this allows your body to effectively improve its top-end performance.

Best for: increased athletic performance, strength gain, general health

ENDURANCE TRAINING: Endurance training is essentially set and rep training, with very high reps per set. If you were performing rows, for example, and your regimen called for five sets of 50 rows, you'd perform 50 rows, take a couple minutes' break, then repeat the row four more times to complete your five sets of 50 reps each.

Endurance training has also been shown to be extremely effective for improving mental health, which is enough by itself to keep endurance training relevant in the changing tides of the exercise science world. Although endurance training doesn't allow you to use as much weight and stimulate your musculature to the same extent as you'd be able to otherwise, it can still help you work toward other goals, if a bit less efficiently. If you prefer the very high-rep nature of endurance training, don't throw it out of your tool belt just because it isn't optimal for physique transformation.

Best for: Increased athletic performance, general health, general conditioning

HIT: High-intensity training is the opposite of eustress training. If eustress training aims to give the body a good workout without overstressing the muscles, HIT aims to tire your muscles out as much as physically possible. It's effective and efficient for a variety of goals, although not necessarily the most enjoyable form of training.

To train in a HIT manner, you simply engage your target muscle continuously until it falters (ideally that would take about 90 seconds). If you wanted to target your quads, for example, you'd perform a wall sit with a sandbag resting on your quads. Ideally, you'd use the correct amount of weight so that your muscles fail after about 90 seconds, give or take 20 seconds either way. If they fail too quickly, then you need to reduce resistance; if they take too long to fail, then you need to increase resistance.

Muscle failure is a very uncomfortable feeling. For HIT training to work, your target muscles must be completely spent after the single set of 70–110 seconds is finished. This means that if you did push-ups to failure, you shouldn't be able to push yourself up off of the ground with your chest muscles until a couple dozen seconds have passed.

Because HIT training is uncomfortable, it isn't for everyone. And it certainly isn't for people working out with the goal of enjoyment. HIT's main virtue is its short time to completion. You can easily get a great workout in less than ten minutes. If you really push yourself and reduce time in between exercises, you can complete an effective workout in less than five minutes.

Best for: fat loss, strength gain, general health

CIRCUIT TRAINING: For the longest time, circuit training was used only by gym classes and athletic teams. When CrossFit rose to prominence, it brought circuit training along for the ride. Circuit training mixes set and rep training with conditioning, making it a fantastic training method for all but those looking to gain mass. It's also a great way to just have a good time moving your body.

Circuit training works like set and rep training, except that there's no rest in between sets and you switch from exercise to exercise after each set. An example of a circuit would be to repeat a cycle of ten push-ups, five pull-ups, and ten lunges five times. Circuits can have as few or as many different exercises as you want, and they can be short or long. One of circuit training's biggest virtues is that it's very flexible, allowing you to shape the workout to your exacting preferences.

Best for: fat loss, increased athletic performance, general health, general conditioning

SCHEDULING YOUR WORKOUTS

Before getting into the actual workouts, let's discuss workout schedules. Although some people prefer to work out whenever motivation strikes, that isn't the best strategy for the vast majority of people. If most of us waited on a whim to work out, our workout consistency would plummet because inaction is usually the default option. When you have a scheduled workout, however, that becomes the default. If you know that you're able to consistently exercise without a set schedule, more power to you. But more than likely you'll need to follow a schedule in order to be consistent and find success with your workout regimen.

There are many different ways to construct a schedule, but there are a few main principles that you should stick to.

1) Schedule your workout at a time that's convenient for you. If it isn't convenient, your consistency and success will suffer.

2) Schedule your workout at a time when your energy levels are fairly high. Our circadian rhythms fluctuate throughout the day, and trying to exercise when you have low energy is a recipe for failure. Working out after lunch, a time when many get sleepy, may not be the best idea.

3) Avoid workouts that put repetitive stress on muscle groups on back-to-back days. Your muscles need time to recover, and not giving them that time can lead to reduced performance and injury. An example of this would be doing bent-over rows on Monday and then pull-ups on Tuesday, which would repetitively stress your back muscles, thus preventing them from full recovery.

With those principles in mind, you now need to construct an actual schedule. Below are a few sample schedules that you can use or modify in a way that better suits your needs. To begin, I suggest you only start with the essentialist workouts, and then add the optional workouts if you want after you've successfully implemented the routine for a month or two. Remember, consistency is the key to results.

SAMPLE WORKOUT SCHEDULES FOR FITNESS GOALS							
	MON	TUE	WED	THU	FRI	SAT	SUN
FAT LOSS	FL 1	rest	FL 2	rest	C 6 (optional)	rest	C 7 (optional)
MUSCLE GAIN	rest	MG 1	rest	MG 2	rest	S&R 2 (optional)	rest
STRENGTH GAIN	SG 1	rest	SG 2	rest	rest	E3 (optional)	rest
INCREASED ATHLETIC PERFORMANCE	IAP 4	IAP 1	EN 10 (optional)	IAP 3	IAP 2	rest	rest
GENERAL HEALTH	GH 1 (optional)	GH 2 (optional)	rest	rest	GH 1	GH 2	rest
GENERAL CONDITIONING	GC 1	GC 2	S&R 1 (optional)	rest	C10 (optional)	rest	rest

For blank templates that you can fill in with your own workout schedule, see page 132.

SAMPLE WORKOUTS

While I can't emphasize enough that an exercise routine is different for every individual, I've created an essentialist workout for each of the most common fitness goals. What is an essentialist workout? It's a workout based on the concept that less is usually better than more. This is also the essence of two very influential books on simplicity: *The ONE Thing* by Gary Keller and *Essentialism* by Greg McKeown. The reason for this is that by paring things down, we spend more time on the essentials, and don't waste time on things that are superfluous.

This is truly applicable to working out. Yes, there are thousands of exercises out there, and thousands of workouts. But if you want to improve efficiently, it makes the most sense to find one or two workouts that are optimally suited to your goal and discard all of the other things that might slow you down. If you have no clue where to begin, give one of these plans a try, tweak them, or discard them completely for your own plan.

I've also compiled few dozen workouts organized by training methods to give you an idea of how to create your own workouts. Feel free to use them exactly as written or adjust them to better fit your needs and desires when creating your weekly workout schedule. You can even mix and match exercises from the workouts. No matter what, remember to tailor your workouts to meet your training goal and fitness level.

Repetitions or time are listed for the exercises, but there's no suggested weight. That's because the weight used is dependent on you. If an exercise lists 10 squats, for example, you should try and find a weight that allows you to perform 10 squats in a row, but not 11. Ideally, as the weeks and months go on you'll be increasing the amount of weight lifted while keeping the reps the same.

ESSENTIALIST WORKOUTS

Best for: *fat loss, muscle gain, strength gain, increased athletic performance, general health, general conditioning*

FAT LOSS

Workout	Exercise	Set x Reps / Duration
FL 1	100-foot Sprint, page 98	20x1
	Burpee, page 106	3x20
FL 2	Sandbag Swing, page 52	3x20
	Push-Up, page 42	3x12
	Inverted Row, page 41	3x8

MUSCLE GAIN

Workout	Exercise	Set x Reps / Duration
MG 1	Back Squat, page 56	4x6
	Chest Press, page 37	4x6
MG 2	Deadlift, page 48	4x6
	Bent-Over Row, page 38	4x6

STRENGTH GAIN

Workout	Exercise	Set x Reps / Duration
SG 1	Front Squat, page 57	10x2
	Chest Press, page 37	10x2
SG 2	Sumo Deadlift, page 50	10x2
	Bent-Over Row, page 38	10x2

IMPROVED ATHLETIC PERFORMANCE

Workout	Exercise	Set x Reps / Duration
IAP 1	Overhead Squat, page 59	12x2
	Push-Up, page 42	12x2
IAP 2	Deadlift, page 48	12x2
	Pull-Up, page 40	12x2
IAP 3	100-foot Sprint, page 98	30x1
	Long Jump, page 118	20x1
	Vertical Jump, page 117	20x1
IAP 4	Sprint, page 98	100 feet
Repeat circuit 50 times	Burpee, page 106	1x3

GENERAL HEALTH		
Workout	Exercise	Set x Reps/Duration
GH 1	Sandbag Swing, page 52	3x20
	Push-Up, page 42	3x12
	Inverted Row, page 41	3x8
GH 2	Distance Ruck, page 119	1 hour
GENERAL CONDITIONING		
Workout	Exercise	Set x Reps/Duration
GC 1	100-foot Sprint, page 98	1x20
	100-foot Shoulder Farmer's Walk, page 103	1x10
GC 2	10-foot Duck Walk, page 85	1x12
	10-foot Crab Walk, page 84	1x12
	10-foot Bear Crawl, page 83	1x12
	10-foot Thruster with Lunge, page 93	1x20

SETS & REPS WORKOUTS

Best for: *fat loss, muscle gain, increased athletic performance, strength gain, general health*

Workout	Exercise	Set x Reps/Duration
S&R 1	Back Squat, page 56	3x5
	Deadlift, page 48	3x5
	Chest Press, page 37	3x5
	Bent-Over Row, page 38	3x5
S&R 2	Wall Sit, page 55	90 seconds
	Push-Up, page 42	3x12
	Pull-Up, page 40	3x5
S&R 3	Front Squat, page 57	5x5
	Chest Press, page 37	5x5
	Calf Raise, page 68	3x10
	Sit-Up, page 75	2x20
S&R 4	Deadlift, page 48	3x5
	Bent-Over Row, page 38	5x5
	Curl, page 46	3x10
	Hand-to-Feet Pass, page 73	2x20
S&R 5	Overhead Squat, page 59	3x8
	Overhead Press, page 34	3x8
	Chest Press, page 37	3x8
	Dip, page 44	3x8
	Calf Raise, page 68	3x10
	Bicycle, page 74	2x20
S&R 6	Sumo Deadlift, page 50	3x8
	Bent-Over Row, page 38	3x8
	Shrug, page 47	3x10
	Skull Crusher, page 45	3x10
	Curl, page 46	3x10
	V-Up, page 76	2x20

S&R 7	Forward Lunge, page 63	4x12 (each leg)
	Muscle-Up, page 39	4x3
	Push Press, page 36	4x12
	Push-Up, page 42	4x12
S&R 8	One-Leg Deadlift, page 49	4x6 (each leg)
	Step-Up, page 65	4x12
	Ground Slam, page 78	4x12
	Chest Toss, page 82	4x12
S&R 9	Clean & Jerk, page 91	5x2
	Snatch, page 90	5x2
	Overhead Chop, page 94	2x20
S&R 10	Turkish Get-Up, page 96	3x6
	Sandbag Swing, page 52	3x24
	Overhead Chop, page 94	2x20

EUSTRESS WORKOUTS

Best for: *increased athletic performance, strength gain, general health*

Workout	Exercise	Set x Reps/Duration
E 1	Back Squat, page 56	30x1
	Chest Press, page 37	30x1
E 2	Deadlift, page 48	30x1
	Bent-Over Row, page 38	30x1
E3	Good Morning, page 61	30x1
	Push-Up, page 42	30x2
	Pull-Up, page 40	30x1
E 4	Front Squat, page 57	30x1
	Dip, page 44	30x1
	Overhead Press, page 34	30x1
	Inverted Row, page 41	30x1
E 5	Top-Heavy Deadlift, page 48	50x1
	One-Arm Overhead Press, page 35	50x1 (each arm)
E 6	One-Leg Deadlift, page 49	50x1 (each leg)
	One-Arm Chest Press, page 37	50x1 (each arm)
E 7	Deadlift, page 48	100x1
E 8	Step-Up, page 65	200x1
E 9	Push-Up, page 42	100x1
E 10	Pull-Up, page 40	50x1

ENDURANCE WORKOUTS

Best for: *Increased athletic performance, general health, general conditioning*

Workout	Exercise	Duration
EN 1	Distance Ruck, page 119	4 hours
EN 2	Stair Ruck, page 120	1 hour
EN 3	Upper-Body Ruck, page 121	20 minutes
EN 4	Deadlift, page 48	5 minutes
	Chest Press, page 37	5 minutes
	Bent-Over Row, page 38	5 minutes
EN 5	Step-Up, page 65	10 minutes (alternating legs)
	Overhead Press, page 34	5 minutes
	Inverted Row, page 41	5 minutes
EN 6	Jumping Rope, page 112	10 minutes
	Sled Pull, page 110	10 minutes
EN 7	Suitcase Farmer's Walk, page 104	20 minutes (switch sides every minute)
EN 8	Overhead Chop, page 94	5 minutes
	Side Chop, page 95	10 minutes (alternating sides)
	Shoveling, page 51	5 minutes
EN 9	Barrel Toss, page 80	10 minutes
	Overhead Throw, page 81	10 minutes
EN 10	Bear Crawl, page 83	5 minutes
	Crab Walk, page 84	5 minutes
	Gorilla Walk, page 86	5 minutes
	Inchworm Walk, page 87	5 minutes
	Army Crawl, page 89	5 minutes
	Duck Walk, page 85	2 minutes

HIT WORKOUTS		
Best for: *fat loss, strength gain, general health*		
Workout	*Exercise*	*Duration*
H 1	Wall Sit, page 55	90 seconds
	Push-Up, page 42	90 seconds
	Pull-Up, page 40	90 seconds
H 2	Static Lunge, page 62	90 seconds (each leg)
	Dip, page 44	90 seconds
	Inverted Row, page 41	90 seconds
H 3	Sumo Squat, page 60	90 seconds
	Overhead Press, page 34	90 seconds
	Bent-Over Row, page 38	90 seconds
H 4	Wall Sit, page 55	90 seconds
	Chest Press, page 37	90 seconds
	Inverted Row, page 41	90 seconds
	Curl, page 46	90 seconds
H 5	One-Leg Wall Sit, page 55	90 seconds (each leg)
	Push-Up, page 42	90 seconds
	Inverted Row, page 41	90 seconds
	Shrug, page 47	90 seconds
H 6	Sumo Squat, page 60	90 seconds
	One-Arm Overhead Press, page 35	90 seconds (each leg)
	One-Arm Bent-Over Row, page 38	90 seconds (each arm)
H 7	Side Lunge, page 64	90 seconds (each leg)
	One-Arm Chest Press, page 37	90 seconds (each arm)
	Pull-Up, page 40	90 seconds
H 8	Wall Sit, page 55	90 seconds
	Push-Up, page 42	90 seconds
	Overhead Press, page 34	90 seconds
	Bent-Over Row, page 38	90 seconds
	Curl, page 46	90 seconds
	Shrug, page 47	90 seconds

H 9	Wall Sit, page 55	90 seconds
	Chest Press, page 37	90 seconds
	Curl, page 46	90 seconds
	Shrug, page 47	90 seconds
H 10	Wall Sit, page 55	90 seconds
	Bent-Over Row, page 38	90 seconds
	Curl, page 46	90 seconds
	Shrug, page 47	90 seconds

CIRCUIT WORKOUTS

Best for: *fat loss, increased athletic performance, general health, general conditioning*

Workout	Exercise	Reps / Duration
C 1	Burpee, page 106	100
C 2	Turkish Get-Up, page 96	100
C 3 *Repeat circuit 5 times*	Burpee, page 106	10
	Turkish Get-Up, page 96	10
C 4 *Repeat circuit 5 times*	Thruster with Lunge, page 93	10 (each leg)
	Jumping Jack, page 111	30
	10-foot Crab Walk, page 84	6
	Sandbag Whip, page 113	30
	High Plank, page 69	1 minute
C 5 *Repeat circuit 10 times*	Front Squat with Arm Extension, page 58	10
	Ground Slam, page 78	10
	10-foot Bear Crawl, page 83	6
	Forearm Plank, page 69	1 minute
C 6 *Repeat circuit 10 times*	Overhead Throw, page 81	10
	Wall Ball, page 79	10
	Barrel Toss, page 80	10
	Box Jump, page 114	10
C 7 *Repeat circuit 15 times*	10-foot Bear Crawl, page 83	2
	10-foot Crab Walk, page 84	2
	10-foot Gorilla Walk, page 86	2
	10-foot Duck Walk, page 85	1
	100-foot Overhead Farmer's Walk, page 105	1
C 8 *Repeat circuit 20 times*	10-foot Inchworm Walk, page 87	2
	10-foot Army Crawl, page 89	1
	100-foot Sprint, page 98	1
	100-foot Overhead Farmer's Walk, page 105	1

C 9	Step-Up, page 65	10 (each leg)
Repeat circuit 15 times	Overhead Chop, page 94	10
	Side Chop, page 95	10 (each side)
	100-foot Side Shuffle Sprint, page 99	1
	100-foot Carioca Sprint, page 100	1
C 10	Vertical Jump, page 117	10
Repeat circuit 10 times	Long Jump, page 118	10
	Rolling Burpee, page 108	10
	Around the World, page 66	10 (each way)
	Shouldering, page 54	10 (each shoulder)

PART 3:
EXERCISES

OVERHEAD PRESS

TARGET: Shoulders

The overhead press develops vertical pushing strength, which doesn't get trained nearly as much as horizontal pushing strength. A completely different set of muscles gets used by this enjoyable but surprisingly difficult movement.

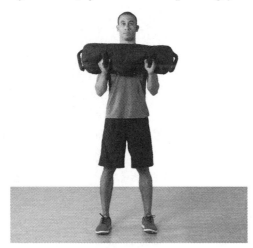

1: Stand with your feet shoulder-width apart and your chest high, roll your shoulders back and down, engage your core, and hold a sandbag at chest level.

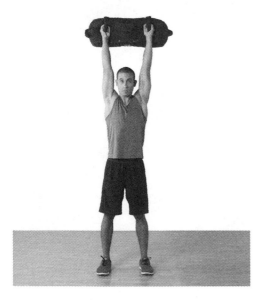

2: Use your arms and shoulders to push the sandbag up until your arms are almost completely extended.

Lower the sandbag back to your chest to complete the rep.

SEATED VARIATION

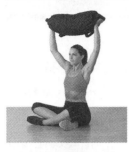

By either sitting or kneeling while pressing, our legs can no longer compensate for a lack of strength in our shoulders and arms.

ONE-ARM VARIATION

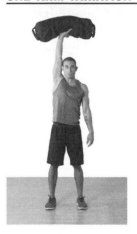

The one-hand overhead press gives the shoulders, arms, and core an extra challenge. (This may require a smaller sandbag.)

PUSH PRESS

TARGET: Shoulders, glutes, quads

If a seated overhead press de-emphasizes the legs, the push press does the opposite and intentionally gives them work. This exercise is a great way to go a bit heavier on the overhead press and allow the body to work from the feet to the shoulders.

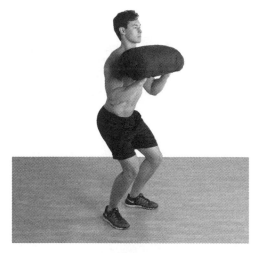

1: Stand with your feet shoulder-width apart and your chest high, roll your shoulders back and down, engage your core, and hold a sandbag at chest level. Squat down two inches.

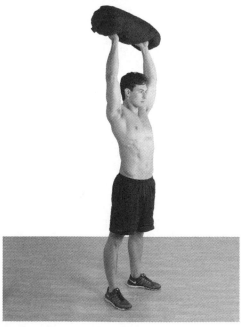

2: Push up through your mid-foot and then use your arms and shoulders to push the sandbag up until arms are almost completely extended.

Lower the sandbag back to your chest to complete the rep.

CHEST PRESS

TARGET: Chest

Though perhaps known as the staple exercise of all fraternity workout plans, the chest press is a great movement for anyone hoping to improve their pushing strength. Using a sandbag for the chest press is more complex than using a barbell, and as a result requires more coordination and engagement from the chest, arms, and hands.

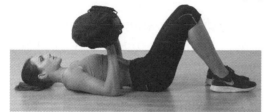

1: Lie on your back with your feet flat on the ground and hold a sandbag an inch above your chest.

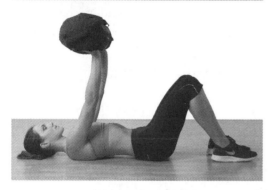

2: Keeping your chest high, roll your shoulders back and down, engage your core, and then use your chest muscles to push the sandbag up until your arms are almost completely extended.

Lower the sandbag to your chest to complete the rep.

ONE-ARM VARIATION

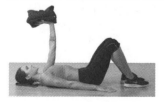

Make the chest press even harder? Use only one hand! The one-hand chest press will test your balance and focus in addition to your strength. (This may require the use of a smaller sandbag.)

INCLINE/DECLINE VARIATION

Mixing the chest press with an incline or decline strengthens your pushing muscles across multiple planes of motion. An angle between 15 degrees and 60 degrees will work. This stimulates different muscles than a flat chest press plus decreases the wear and tear on joints that would have to otherwise repeatedly go through the exact same range of motion.

BENT-OVER ROW

TARGET: Lats, back

The bent-over row is a straightforward, effective, and fun way to build pulling strength. Not only do the back muscles get heavy work but the whole posterior chain has to be active in order to perform the movement correctly. Sandbags with handles also lend themselves very well to the bent-over row.

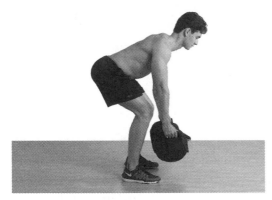

1: Stand with your feet shoulder-width apart and your chest high, roll your shoulders back and down, engage your core, and hold the sandbag by the handles. If your sandbag has no handles, put your hands under the bag to get a solid hold of it. Keep your knees over your ankles, your weight over your mid-foot, and then hinge at the hips until your chest is at a 135-degree angle with the ground.

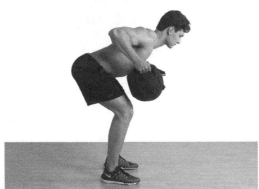

2: Being sure to keep your chest high and your shoulders back and down, use your back to pull the bag toward your chest until your hands reach your torso. Your shoulder blades should feel like they're being pulled together.

Lower the sandbag back toward the ground until your arms are nearly extended to complete the rep.

ONE-ARM VARIATION

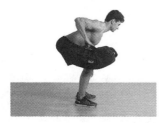

To further involve the posterior chain and the core, try using just one hand for your bent-over rows. Though it doubles the amount of time necessary to do the same amount of work, the one-hand bent-over row is a worthy variation for those looking to strengthen their back muscles. Handles are necessary for this movement.

MUSCLE-UP

TARGET: Lats, back, chest, triceps

Muscle-ups take serious strength.

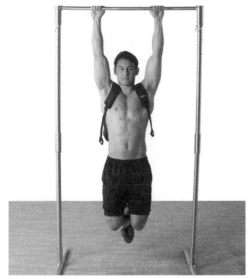

1: Place your hands shoulder-width apart on the bar with the palms of your hands facing away from you. Keep a high chest, roll your shoulders back and down, and engage your core.

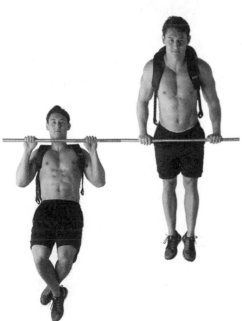

2–3: Starting with arms almost completely extended, pull down on the bar with your back muscles until your chin reaches bar level. Quickly transition your grip for a dip by sliding the heels of your hands on top of the bar and then pushing yourself up over the bar until your arms are almost completely extended.

Smoothly lower yourself back down to starting position to complete the rep.

PULL-UP

TARGET: Lats, back

There is something about pulling your bodyweight over a bar that just feels good.

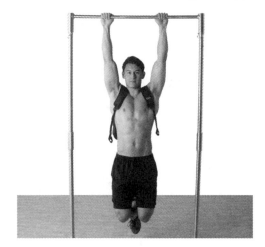

1: Place your hands shoulder-width apart on the bar with the palms of your hands facing away from you. Keep your chest high, roll your shoulders back and down, and engage your core. Your arms are almost completely extended.

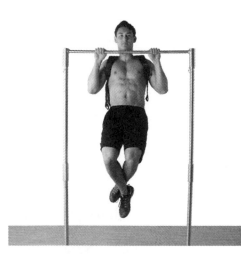

2: Pull down on the bar with your back muscles until your chin reaches bar-level.

Lower yourself back down until your arms are almost fully extended to complete the rep. If full reps are too difficult, reduce the range of motion.

PALMS-FACING VARIATION

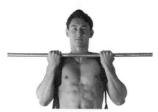

To engage different muscles, perform the pull-up with your palms facing you. Many people also find that this grip makes the movement a bit easier.

ONE-ARM VARIATION

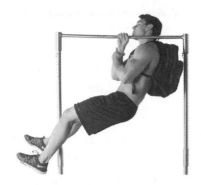

For the ultimate challenge, perform the pull-up with one arm instead of two. To work up to this high-level movement, reduce the number of fingers used by one hand to strengthen the opposite arm until you're able to perform a pull-up with just one arm.

INVERTED ROW VARIATION

Inverted rows are a great movement for those not quite able to bang out full pull-ups. Even for those that can do full pull-ups, adding weight with a sandbag allows you to make inverted rows as difficult as any other pulling movement.

1: Secure a weighted backpack on your back and then grab onto the rings or handles dangling vertically. Lower yourself down until your shoulders are directly below the rings or handles. Keep your feet neutral, with the weight on your heels. Keep your body as straight as possible and your chest high, roll your shoulders back and down, and engage your core.

2: Use your back to smoothly pull yourself up until your hands reach your torso. Your shoulder blades should feel like they're being pulled together. Smoothly lower yourself back down until your arms are almost completely extended to complete the rep.

PUSH-UP

TARGET: Chest, triceps

Perhaps the most common resistance exercise in the world, the push-up is easily adjusted to be easy or difficult, can be done anywhere with no extra equipment, and engages the whole body from head to toe.

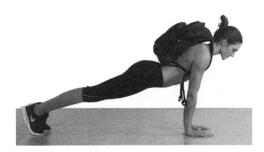

1: Place sandbags in a backpack and wear the backpack on your back. Get on all four limbs with your hands directly below your shoulders and your arms almost completely extended. Keep your chest high, roll your shoulders back and down, and engage your core.

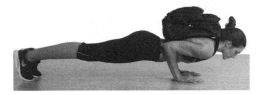

2: Keeping your back straight in a line that gently slopes from toes to head, use your chest and arms to smoothly lower yourself down until your chest is an inch off the ground.

At the bottom of the movement, push yourself up until your arms are almost completely extended to complete the rep.

KNEE VARIATION

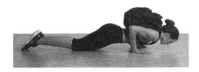

If a normal push-up is too difficult, perform the exercise on your knees.

WIDE/NARROW GRIP VARIATION

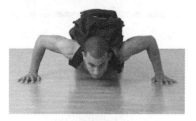

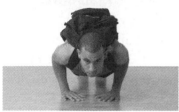

To engage different muscles and challenge your body in a new way, try performing push-ups with your hands closer together or farther apart than shoulder-width.

DIP

TARGET: Chest, triceps

Dips are an effective way to strengthen the pushing muscles through another plane of motion.

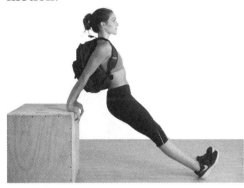

1: Place sandbags in a backpack and wear the backpack on your back. Place your hands on the edge of a sturdy bench or chair with your arms almost completely extended. Keep a high chest, roll your shoulders back and down, and engage your core.

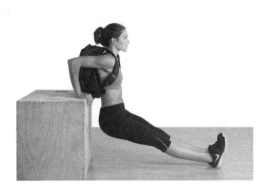

2: Smoothly lower yourself down until your elbows bend roughly 90 degrees.

Push yourself back to starting position with your arms, chest, and back to complete the rep.

MODIFICATION

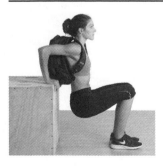

You can also bend your knees.

SKULL CRUSHER

TARGET: Triceps

A solid accessory lift, the skull crusher is one of the most effective ways to target the triceps.

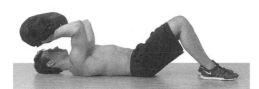

1: Lie on your back with your feet flat on the ground. Keep a high chest, roll your shoulders down and back, engage your core, and start with the sandbag held an inch away from your forehead.

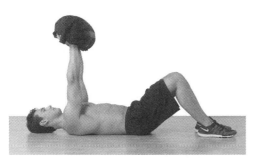

2: Lift the bag by straightening your arms until they're almost completely extended.

Smoothly reverse the motion until the bag is back in its starting position to complete the rep.

CURL

TARGET: Biceps

The curl is an exercise that's commonly utilized by those seeking muscular biceps but also criticized by those who only seek functional strength. There's nothing wrong with this guilty pleasure, though. Do *you* have tickets to the gun show yet?

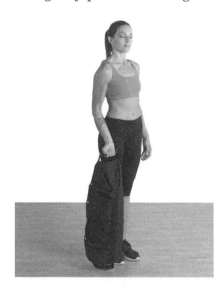

1: Stand with your feet shoulder-width apart and your chest high, roll your shoulders back and down, engage your core, and grab hold of the sandbag's handles or put your hand under the bag if there are none.

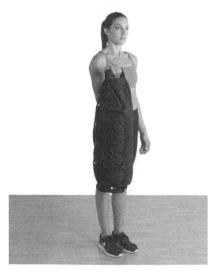

2: Curl the bag 180 degrees, until your forearm is perpendicular to the ground.

Smoothly reverse the motion until the bag is returned to its starting position to complete the rep.

SHRUG

TARGET: Traps

The shrug is a move mainly used by bodybuilders, but it's a decent accessory lift for anyone who wants to target the upper traps. If it was the move used by Atlas, it must be effective....

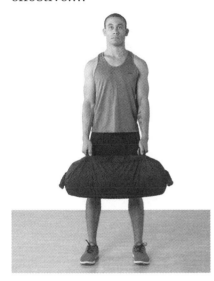

1: Stand with your feet shoulder-width apart and your chest high, roll your shoulders back and down, engage your core, and hold the sandbag by its handles, or grip the sandbag by its extra fabric if there are none.

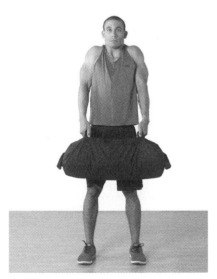

2: To move the sandbag up, shrug your shoulders up toward your ears until they're as high as they can go.

Smoothly lower your shoulders down until they return to their neutral starting position to complete the rep.

DEADLIFT

TARGET: Glutes, hamstrings

Although squats get a lot of functional training attention, the deadlift may transfer even better to day-to-day life. Not only does it increase our ability to lift things off the ground, it may also be the single most effective resistance exercise to increase sprint speed.

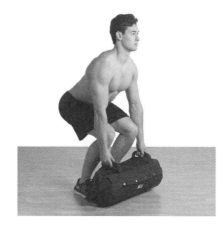

1: Stand with your feet shoulder-width apart and your chest high, keep a very slight bend in your knees, roll your shoulders back and down, and engage your core. Hinge at the hips to pick the sandbag up by the handles or by getting your hands under the sandbag, being sure to keep a high chest throughout the movement.

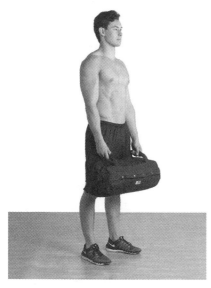

2: Using your glutes and hamstrings, pull the sandbag up from the ground until you resume the standing position.

Smoothly reverse the motion and set the sandbag down to complete the rep.

TOP-HEAVY VARIATION

Hold the sandbag tightly against your chest instead of holding it with extended arms.

ONE-LEG DEADLIFT

TARGET: Glutes, hamstrings

The one-leg deadlift requires more concentration and balance than the two-legged deadlift, making it a good choice for athletes or anyone up for a challenge. It isn't an easy movement, though, so be sure to put extra emphasis on proper form and use a much lighter weight.

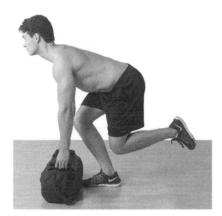

1: Stand with your feet shoulder-width apart and your chest high, keep a very slight bend in your knees, roll your shoulders back and down, and engage your core. Lift one foot off of the ground and hinge at the hips to pick the sandbag up by the handles or by getting your hands under the sandbag, being sure to keep a high chest throughout the movement.

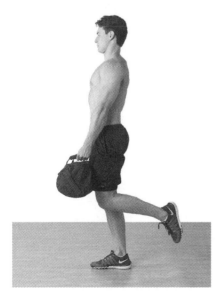

2: Using your glutes and hamstrings, pull the sandbag up from the ground until you resume the standing position.

Smoothly reverse the motion and set the sandbag down to complete the rep.

Repeat, and then switch legs.

SUMO DEADLIFT

TARGET: Glutes, hamstrings

For a twist on the traditional deadlift, move your feet farther apart and give the sumo deadlift a try. But be careful: The farther away your feet are from each other, the greater the range of motion you'll need from your hamstrings.

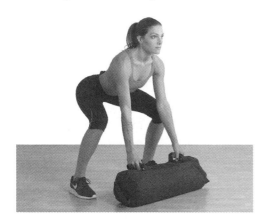

1: Stand with your feet shoulder-width apart and your chest high, keep a very slight bend in your knees, roll your shoulders back and down, and engage your core. Hinge at the hips to pick the sandbag up by the handles or by getting your hands under the sandbag.

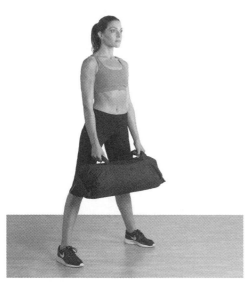

2: Keeping a high chest throughout the movement, use your glutes and hamstrings to pull the sandbag up from the ground until you resume the standing position.

Smoothly reverse the motion and set the sandbag down to complete the rep.

SHOVELING

TARGET: Glutes, hamstrings

In a world where the kettlebell swing has taken off, sandbag shoveling should also be destined for exercise stardom. It's a great movement that targets the always-essential hip hinge in a realistic way. Gain back some functional strength with sandbag shoveling!

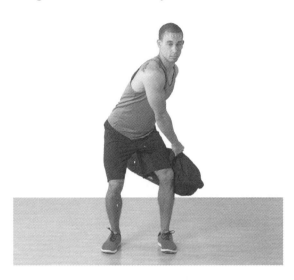

1: Stand with your feet shoulder-width apart and your chest high, roll your shoulder blades back and down, and engage your core. Hold the sandbag by the handles or get a secure grip underneath the sandbag. Start with the sandbag to the side of your knee.

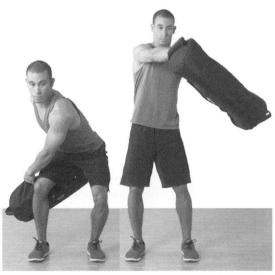

2–3: Use the leg closest to the sandbag and your core to smoothly swing the sandbag to the side of your other knee. Your glutes should be doing a large portion of the work, and your back should be straight, not rounded. As soon as the sandbag gets to the side of your other knee, use that leg to swing the sandbag back to the other knee.

Continue the fluid movement without stopping until your desired amount of reps is reached.

SANDBAG SWING

TARGET: Glutes, hamstrings

Though perhaps not as graceful to swing as kettlebells, sandbags are just as effective. Few exercises allow for the combination of work rate and work weight that the swing provides, which is the reason it's so effective at both building strength and endurance.

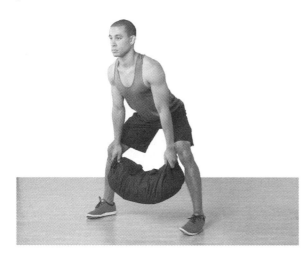

1: Stand with your feet wider than shoulder-width apart and your chest high, roll your shoulder blades back and down, and engage your core. Hinge at the hips and grip the sandbag by the handles.

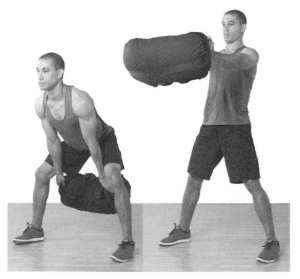

2–3: Swing the sandbag back a few inches. Then immediately push the bag forward with your glutes and hamstrings.

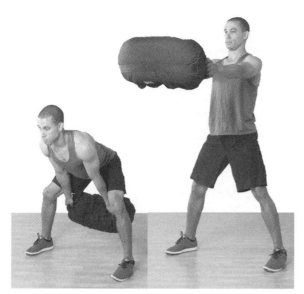

4–5: Without any pause, allow the bag to swing back between your legs and then use your legs to push the bag up to chest level.

Continue this two-step process until you complete your desired amount of reps.

To end the movement, use your glutes and hamstrings to smoothly slow down the momentum of the bag.

SHOULDERING

TARGET: Glutes, hamstrings

Shouldering can only really be done with a sandbag, making it a staple among sandbag trainers in the know. Cadence can be fast for light weights and slow for heavy weights.

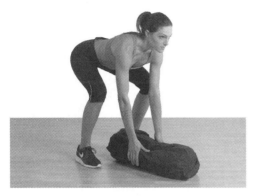

1: Stand with your feet shoulder-width apart and your chest high, roll your shoulder blades back and down, and engage your core. With the sandbag between your legs on the ground, hinge at the hips (being sure to keep a straight back and high hips) and grab hold of the sandbag.

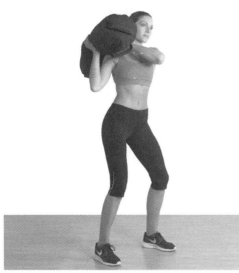

2: Smoothly explode up with the sandbag, using your glutes and hamstrings to bring the sandbag onto your shoulder.

With a tight core and posterior chain lower the sandbag to the ground to complete the rep. Switch shoulders every rep.

WALL SIT

TARGET: Quads

The wall sit builds quad strength as well as mental strength.

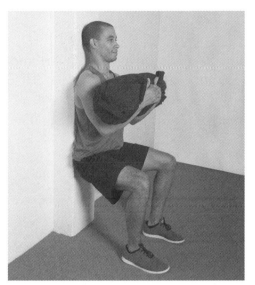

THE POSITION: Lean against a wall so your back is flat and your legs make a 90-degree angle. Hold a sandbag in a bear hug or rest it on your quads. Keep that posture until your desired amount of time is up.

ONE-LEG VARIATION

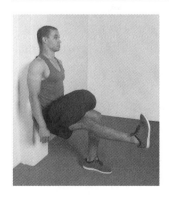

Do weighted wall sits not provide enough of a challenge? Pick one leg off the floor! An added bonus of the one-leg wall sit is that it can help you progress toward the challenge of completing a pistol squat. Switch legs after the first leg tires out.

BACK SQUAT

TARGET: Glutes, quads

The back squat is a go-to exercise for football players, distance runners, and pretty much anyone else who wants a stronger set of legs. Why? Because it allows for the use of heavy weight and is a total-body, functional exercise.

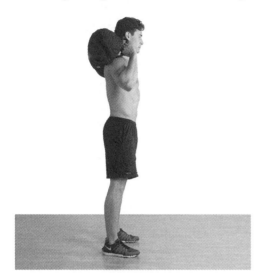

1: Stand with your feet shoulder-width apart and your chest high, roll your shoulder blades back and down, and engage your core. Hoist the sandbag onto the top of your back, right below your neck.

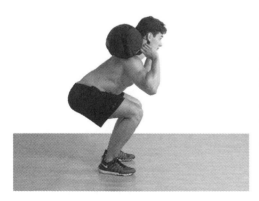

2: Break at the hips and slowly bring them back and down. Your knees will naturally start to bend. Fight to keep a high chest, don't allow your knees to move inward, and be sure to engage your glutes. Go down as far as you can, but stop before your back starts to round. Your back should stay straight throughout the movement.

Once you've reached your lowest point, push down through your mid-foot until you reach your starting position to complete the rep.

FRONT SQUAT

TARGET: Glutes, quads

The front squat lends itself a bit better to the sandbag modality, and is a very worthy alternative to the back squat. It's also much more functional since, in real life, we tend to hold things in front of our bodies rather than behind them.

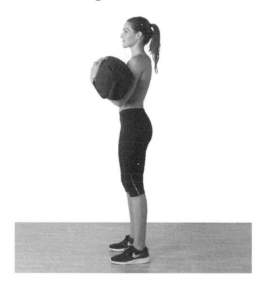

1: Stand with your feet shoulder-width apart and your chest high, roll your shoulder blades back and down, and engage your core. Hold the sandbag against your chest in a bear hug or press it against your chest horizontally so it rests on your biceps.

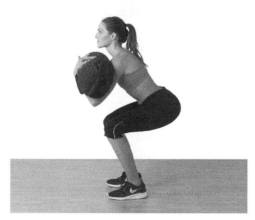

2: Break at the hips and slowly bring them back and down. Your knees will naturally start to bend. Fight to keep a high chest, don't allow your knees to move inward, and be sure to engage your glutes. Go down as far as you can, but stop before your back starts to round. Your back should stay straight throughout the movement.

Once you've reached your lowest point, push down through your mid-foot until you reach your starting position to complete the rep.

FRONT SQUAT WITH ARM EXTENSION

TARGET: Glutes, quads, shoulders, biceps

Adding the arm extension to the front squat means you're also giving your core and arms a good workout.

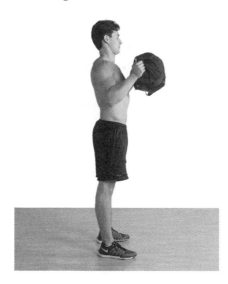

1: Stand with your feet shoulder-width apart and your chest high, roll your shoulders back and down, and engage your core. Start with the sandbag at your chest.

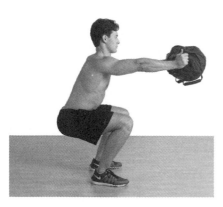

2: Squat down with your arms extending forward as you descend. Your arms should be almost fully extended at the bottom of your squat.

Squat back up to starting position with your arms bringing the sandbag in as you rise to complete the rep.

OVERHEAD SQUAT

TARGET: Glutes, quads, shoulders

The overhead squat is not only a great exercise to improve leg strength, but it also helps with squatting form, something that most of us in the sitting-centric developed world need to improve upon. Holding a sandbag overhead forces us to have a very strong core. You'll have to really fight to keep a high chest and arms that go straight up.

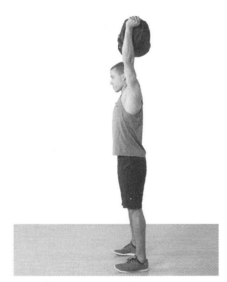

1: Stand with your feet shoulder-width apart and your chest high, roll your shoulder blades back and down, and engage your core. Hold the sandbag directly overhead with your arms almost completely extended.

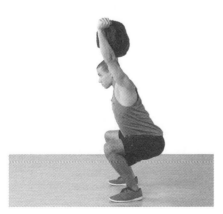

2: Break at the hips and slowly bring them back and down. Your knees will naturally start to bend. Fight to keep a high chest, don't allow your knees to move inward, and be sure to engage your glutes. Go down as far as you can, but stop before your back starts to round. Your back should stay straight throughout the movement.

Once you've reached your lowest point, push down through your mid-foot until you reach your starting position to complete the rep.

SUMO SQUAT

TARGET: Glutes, quads

Add the sumo squat to your workout if you want to mix things up without eliminating the all-important squat altogether.

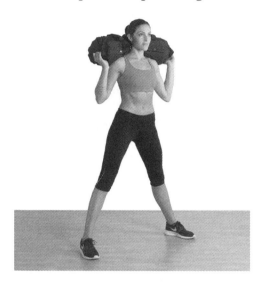

1: Stand with your feet wider than shoulder-width apart and your chest high, roll your shoulder blades back and down, and engage your core. Hoist the sandbag onto the top of your back, right below your neck.

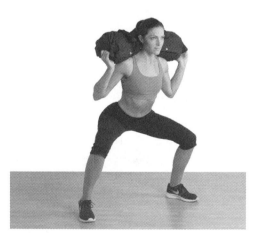

2: Break at the hips and slowly bring them back and down. Your knees will naturally start to bend. Fight to keep a high chest, don't allow your knees to move inward, and be sure to engage your glutes. Go down as far as you can, but stop before your back starts to round. Your back should stay straight throughout the movement.

Once you've reached your lowest point, push down through your mid-foot until you reach your starting position to complete the rep.

GOOD MORNING

TARGET: Glutes, hamstrings, back

Good mornings target your posterior-chain muscles. They make a great stand-in if you want to take a break from deadlifts, or can be a simple, effective addition to any workout.

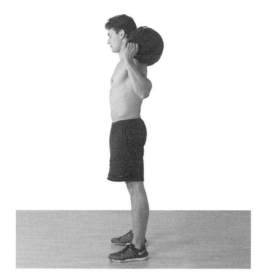

1: Stand with your feet shoulder-width apart and your chest high, keep a very slight bend in the knees, and roll your shoulders back and down while engaging your core. Hoist the sandbag onto your upper back, right below your neck.

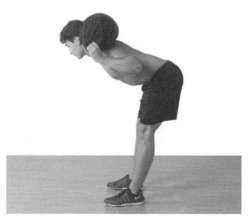

2: Without moving your legs, hinge at the hips and come down as far as your hamstrings will allow. Be sure to keep a high chest and straight back.

After reaching the bottom of your range of motion, without moving your legs, use your glutes and hamstrings to return to starting position to complete the rep.

STATIC LUNGE

TARGET: Glutes, quads

Static lunges demand near-constant muscle engagement, a great way to give your legs a lot of work in a short time.

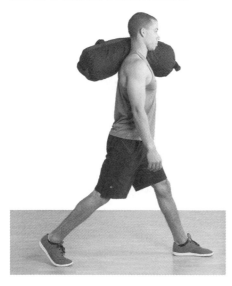

1: Hoist the sandbag onto one shoulder. With a high chest, roll your shoulders down and back, engage your core, and take a step forward.

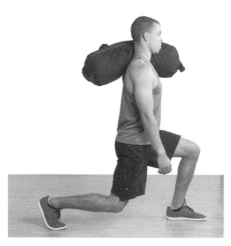

2: Using your glutes and quads, lower yourself down until your leg makes a 90-degree angle, keeping your ankle directly under your knee.

Smoothly use the same muscles to push yourself back up through the mid-foot to complete the rep. Keep your feet on the ground in the same place throughout the exercise. Repeat with the same leg until your target number of reps are completed, and then switch the sandbag to the other shoulder and use your other leg.

FORWARD LUNGE

TARGET: Glutes, quads

This versatile lunge can be done with heavy weight, no weight at all, inside, or outside. It's also likely to help you reach your training goals, whether they're to improve athletic performance, put on weight, or lose it.

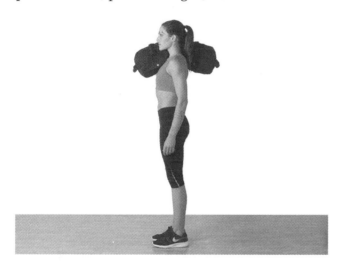

1: Hoist the sandbag onto one shoulder. With a high chest, roll your shoulders down and back, and engage your core.

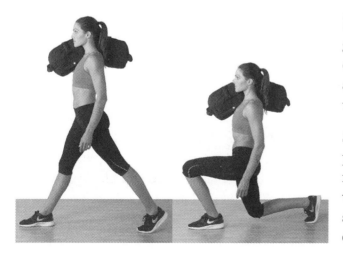

2–3: Take a step forward and use your glutes and quads to lower yourself down until your leg makes a 90-degree angle, keeping your ankle directly under your knee.

Smoothly use the same muscles to push yourself back up through the mid-foot to complete the rep. Repeat with the other leg, and switch the sandbag to the other shoulder after each set.

SIDE LUNGE

TARGET: Glutes, quads

The side lunge is just as effective as the front lunge but engages different muscles, making it a great addition or replacement for the lunge. As far as sports enhancement goes, the side lunge transfers especially well to basketball or any sport that emphasizes side-to-side movement.

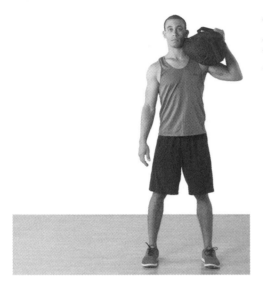

1: Hoist the sandbag onto your shoulder. With a high chest, roll your shoulders down and back, and engage your core.

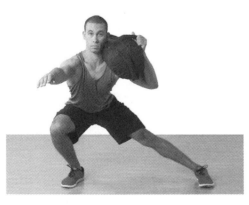

2: Take a step sideways and use your glutes and quads to lower yourself down until your leg makes a 90-degree angle, keeping your ankle directly under your knee.

Smoothly use the same muscles to push yourself back up through the mid-foot to complete the rep. Repeat with the other leg, and switch the sandbag to the other shoulder after each set.

STEP-UP

TARGET: Glutes, quads

The step-up is a safe, simple movement for building leg strength. It can be easily modified for endurance or strength goals by adding small or large amounts of weight.

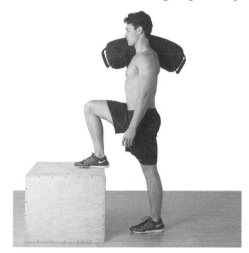

1: Hoist a sandbag onto your shoulder with a high chest. Roll your shoulders back and down, and engage your core. Step onto a 12- to 24-inch platform with your ankle directly below your knee.

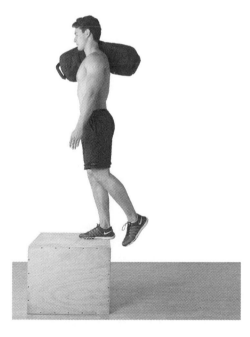

2: Use your glutes, quads, and hamstrings to push through the mid-foot and raise your body up until it's completely upright on the platform.]

Slowly lower yourself down to starting position and repeat the movement with the other leg. Switch the sandbag to the other shoulder after each set.

AROUND THE WORLD

TARGET: Abs

The around the world looks cool and is lots of fun. It's also a very effective exercise for increasing core strength in addition to being useful for endurance conditioning.

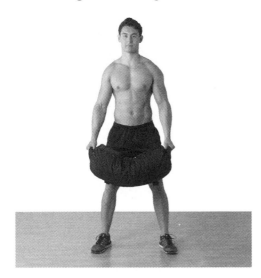

1: Stand with your feet shoulder-width apart and your chest high, roll your shoulders back and down, and engage your core. Hold the sandbag by its handles or by gripping the bag's fabric if there are none, allowing it to hang in front of your legs.

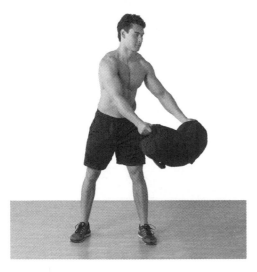

2: Use your whole body to swing the sandbag quickly to your side.

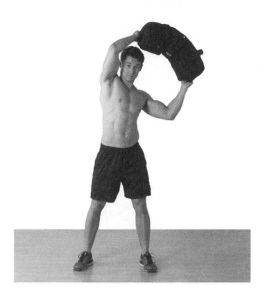

3: Use the sandbag's momentum to swing it around your head. The sandbag's momentum will bring it back to its original position in the center of your body.

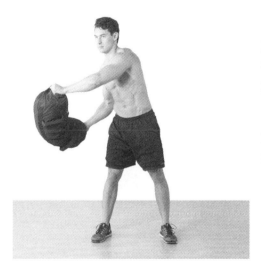

4: Rather than slowing the sandbag down, use your legs, core, and arms to continue to sandbag's movement, completing another circle around your head.

Continue this cycle until your desired number of reps is reached, and then complete the movement in the other direction.

CALF RAISE

TARGET: Calves

Whether you want to jump higher for athletics or just build muscular calves, the calf raise is a very reasonable accessory lift. Be sure to go through the whole range of motion!

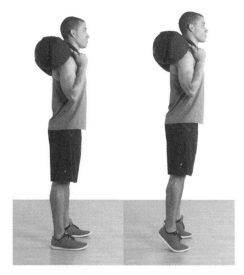

1–2: Stand with your feet shoulder-width apart and your chest high, roll your shoulders back and down, and engage your core. Hold the sandbag by the handles, in a bear hug, or on your shoulder. Press the balls of your feet into the ground and raise your heels off the ground as high as they can go.

Smoothly return to starting position to complete the rep.

SEATED VARIATION

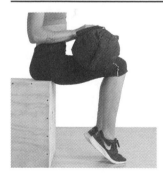

If you want to grab a breather after a set of sprints or heavy squats, go for some seated calf raises with the sandbag resting on your thighs. Some people also just prefer them to standing calf raises.

FOREARM PLANK

TARGET: Abs

Ah, the plank—a favorite of youth athletic coaches around the world, and for good reason. Planking helps increase core stability and mental strength.

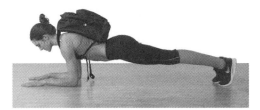

THE POSITION: Place sandbags in a backpack and wear it on your back. Place your forearms flat on the ground so that your elbows are directly under your shoulders. Extend your legs behind you, keeping your legs three inches apart and the balls of your feet on the ground. Your back should form a straight line from head to heels. Keep this posture until the desired amount of time passes.

HIGH PLANK

TARGET: Abs

More challenging than the forearm version, the high plank is a great core exercise to mix in any workout.

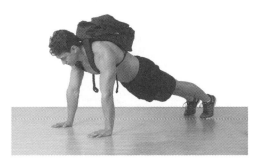

THE POSITION: Place sandbags in a backpack and wear it on your back. Place your hands on the ground so that they're directly under your shoulders. Extend your legs behind you, keeping your legs three inches apart and the balls of your feet on the ground. Your back should form a straight line from head to heels. Keep this posture until the desired amount of time passes.

SIDE PLANK

TARGET: Abs

The side plank targets core muscles seldom worked. It's often recommended to athletes and those trying to reduce nagging back pain.

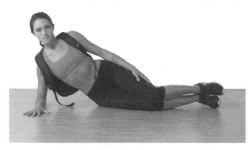

1: Place sandbags in a backpack and wear it on your back. Lie on your side with your elbow directly under your shoulder.

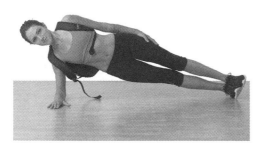

2: Keeping a completely straight torso and your hips, shoulders, and feet stacked atop each other, push yourself up so that the only things touching the ground are your forearm and your foot.

Keep this posture until the desired amount of time passes.

VARIATION

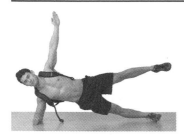

To make the exercise more difficult, you can raise and lower your top arm and leg as if you were doing a jumping jack.

REVERSE PLANK

TARGET: Back

The reverse plank is a worthy addition to your core routine, and is a good stepping stone to the more difficult glute-ham plank (below).

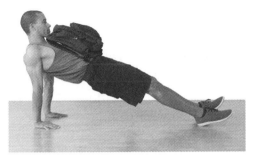

THE POSITION: Place sandbags in a backpack and wear it on your front. Sit on the floor with your hands on the ground and fingers pointing at your butt; your hands should be directly under your shoulders, pressing your weight into your hands and your heels, lift your butt off the ground until your body makes a straight line from your feet to your shoulders.

Keep this posture until the desired amount of time passes.

GLUTE-HAM PLANK

TARGET: Glutes, hamstrings, back

The glute-ham plank is the most underrated member of the plank family. It's the best at strengthening the all-important posterior chain, however, which is crucial in preventing back issues.

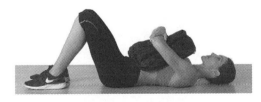

1: Hugging a sandbag to your chest, lie on your back with your knees slightly bent, feet on the ground, and feet and knees together.

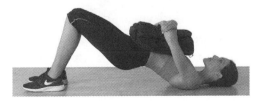

2: Push your heels into the ground with your glutes and hamstrings to raise your glutes and lower back off the ground two inches.

Keep this posture until the desired amount of time passes.

BIRD DOG

TARGET: Abs

The bird dog is an awesome core exercise, one that I use frequently to stave off nagging back pain. It's also a good way to make sure your core is engaged before a workout.

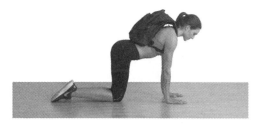

1: Place sandbags in a backpack and wear it on your back. Get on all fours, with your knees on the ground directly under your hips and your hands on the ground directly below your shoulders, arms almost completely extended. Keep a completely straight back.

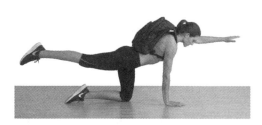

2: Without twisting your pelvis/hips, smoothly extend your right arm forward and left leg backward.

Bring them right back in to complete the rep and then switch to your left arm and right leg.

SUPERMAN

TARGET: Glutes, hamstrings, back

The superman excels at strengthening the posterior chain.

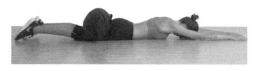

1: Lie on your stomach and place the sandbag on your hamstrings, right above the backs of your knees.

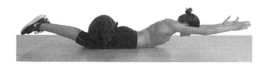

2: Bend your knees, extend your arms, and bring all limbs off the ground about an inch. Focus on keeping continuous stability from your heels to your neck.

Hold this posture until the desired time passes.

HAND-TO-FEET PASS

TARGET: Abs

In the never-ending quest to keep core exercises fresh, hand-to-feet passes are nice because they allow you to concentrate on the movement of the sandbag rather than the burning sensation of your abs.

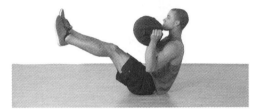

1: With the sandbag in your hands, sit on the ground with your arms and legs off the ground.

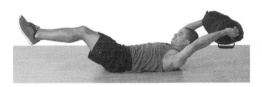

2: Slowly extend your arms behind your head and lower your legs toward the ground. Stop your descent as your arms and legs are fully extended and an inch from the ground.

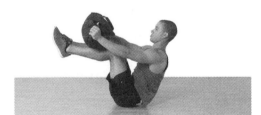

3: Sit back up and transfer the sandbag to your legs.

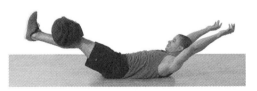

4: Perform the same movement back down and up to complete the rep.

BICYCLE

TARGET: Abs

If you wanted to include one abdominal exercise in a workout, ab bicycles would be a fine choice. They're effective but not particularly enjoyable.

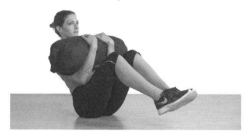

1: Sit on the ground with your legs off the ground. Hold the sandbag in your arms.

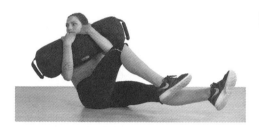

2: Twist to touch your left elbow to your right knee.

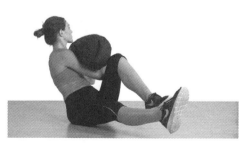

3: To complete the rep, twist the other way to touch your right elbow to your left knee.

Switch arms after every set.

SIT-UP

TARGET: Abs

Incorporating sandbags into sit-ups nearly makes you forget about how they plagued you in gym class. Though sit-ups have gotten a bad rap in the last couple of decades, they still remain an effective core training tool.

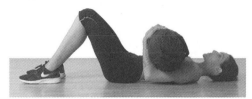

1: Lie on your back with your knees bent and your feet flat on the ground. Hold the sandbag at your chest or an inch above your head.

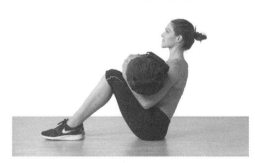

2: Use your core to bring your chest up to your knees.

Smoothly lower yourself back down to the ground to complete the rep.

V-UP

TARGET: Abs

If regular sit-ups are too easy, try V-ups.

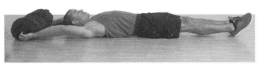

1: Lie on your back with your arms and legs almost completely extended. Hold the sandbag in your hands.

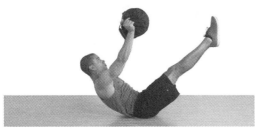

2: Keeping your core fully engaged and your arms and legs almost completely extended, raise your feet and hands until your lower back and hamstrings are both off the ground.

Smoothly return to starting position to complete the rep.

VARIATION

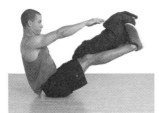

You can also try holding the sandbag between your feet.

FROZEN V

TARGET: Abs

For the masochists that relish the burn of isometric movements, the frozen V is for you.

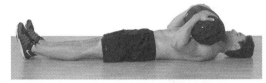

1: Lie on your back with your arms and legs almost completely extended. Hold the sandbag in your hands.

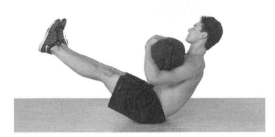

2: Keeping your core fully engaged and your arms and legs almost completely extended, raise your feet and hands until your lower back and hamstrings are both off the ground. Hold the position until your desired amount of time has passed.

GROUND SLAM

TARGET: Glutes, abs, shoulders, triceps

Throwing a tantrum is fun, but who knew it could be such a good workout? Ground slams allow you to unleash all of your pent-up feelings yet result in a strengthened core instead of a timeout.

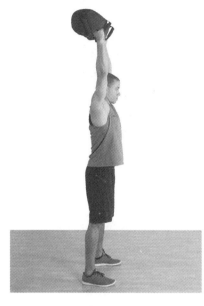

1: Stand with your feet shoulder-width apart and your chest high, roll your shoulders down and back, and engage your core. Hinge at the hips and hoist the sandbag above your head.

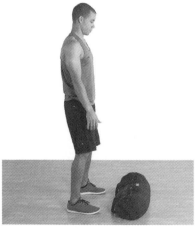

2: Use your core, shoulders, and arms to throw the bag down in front of you to complete the rep.

WALL BALL

TARGET: Glutes, quads, chest, shoulders

Playing wall ball by yourself has never been this fun or productive. You'll get a killer full-body workout, varying the weight used to favor strength or endurance.

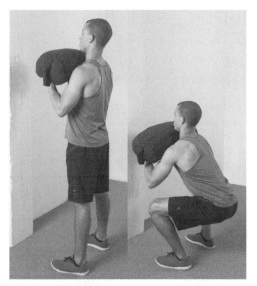

1–2: Stand a foot away from a very sturdy wall with your feet shoulder-width apart, your chest high, your shoulders rolled down and back, and your core engaged. Hold the sandbag at your chest as you would a basketball before throwing a chest pass. Lower down for a full squat.

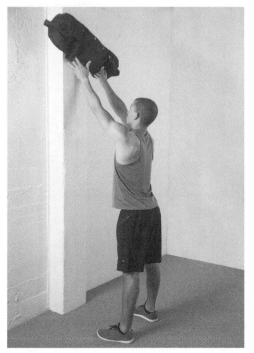

3: Explode up with your legs, and keep the sandbag's momentum going by extending your arms and throwing the sandbag at the wall one foot above your head.

Catch the sandbag on its way down before continuing the motion by squatting again and then throwing the sandbag against the wall.

BARREL TOSS

TARGET: Glutes, hamstrings, shoulders

If you've ever watched *World's Strongest Man*, you've probably wanted to give the barrel toss a try. Now you can without being, well, one of the world's strongest men.

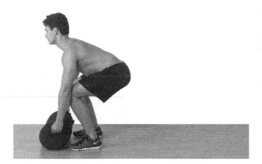

1: Stand with your feet shoulder-width apart and your chest high, roll your shoulders back and down, and engage your core. Hinge at the hips with the sandbag in front of you and grab hold of the bag.

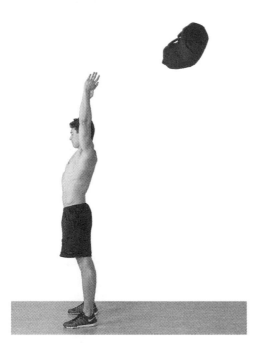

2: In a smooth but explosive movement, use your glutes, hamstrings, and back to throw the bag over your head backward as far as you can.

OVERHEAD THROW

TARGET: Abs, shoulders, triceps

In addition to being sport-specific training for soccer and basketball, the overhead throw is an explosive movement that targets the core and arms.

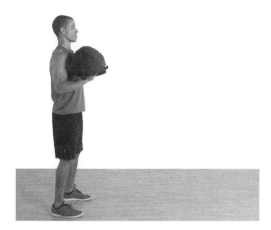

1: Stand with your feet shoulder-width apart and your chest high, roll your shoulders down and back, and engage your core. Hold the sandbag at chest level.

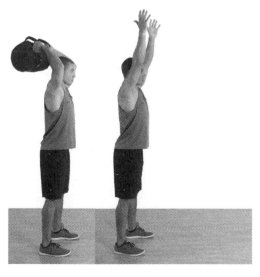

2–3: Bring the sandbag over your head, and then use your core and arms to throw the bag forward as far as you can.

CHEST TOSS

TARGET: Chest, shoulders

The chest toss targets the chest, making it a great addition to workouts aimed at increasing pushing strength. It's fun but requires a lower weight than you may anticipate in order to engage the chest instead of the shoulders.

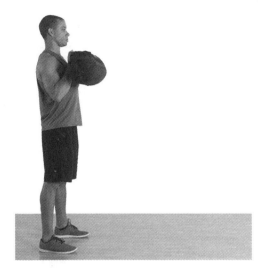

1: Stand with your feet shoulder-width apart and your chest high, roll your shoulders down and back, and engage your core. Hold the sandbag at chest level.

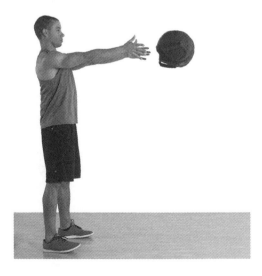

2: Use your core and chest to explosively push the sandbag away from your chest, throwing it as far as you can.

BEAR CRAWL

TARGET: Chest, shoulders, abs

The bear crawl trains your hips to stay high and powerful, which is helpful for athletics and day-to-day life. It's also an exercise that can be done at a high intensity, lending itself very well to conditioning work.

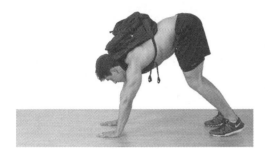

1: Place sandbags in a backpack and wear it on your back. Place your hands on the ground, keeping your weight evenly distributed between your hands and the balls of your feet.

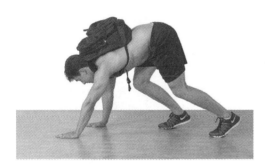

2: With your hips a bit higher than your chest and your back straight, move your left hand and right leg forward.

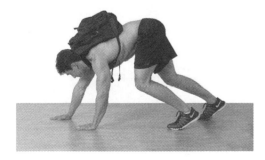

3: Continue this motion by moving your right hand and left foot forward.

Keep crawling until your desired distance or time has been met.

CRAB WALK

TARGET: Back, triceps, shoulders, quads, glutes

When it comes to core stabilization, we spend most of our time with our chest to the ground. The crab walk is a great exercise to mix things up and practice keeping our posterior chain tight through a dynamic movement.

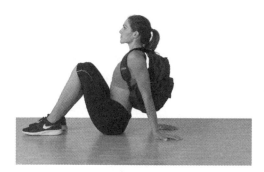

1: Place sandbags in a backpack and wear it on your front. With your stomach facing up, place your hands on the ground and fingers pointing backward. Keep your weight evenly distributed between your hands and heels.

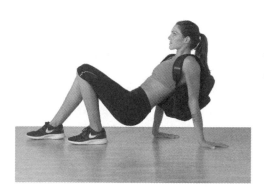

2: With your glutes a few inches off the ground and fingers pointing backward, move one hand and one foot backward.

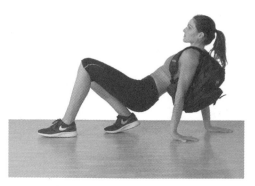

3: Continue this motion by moving your other hand and foot backward.

Keep crawling until your desired distance or time has been met.

DUCK WALK

TARGET: Quads

Battling the wall sit for "most brutal quad exercise" is the duck walk. Who would've thought imitating an animal with such skinny limbs would be such an effective method for building powerful legs?

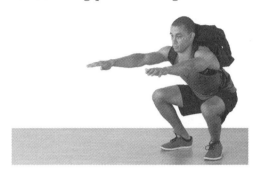

1: Place sandbags in a backpack and wear it on your back. Squat down until your hamstrings are resting on your calves. Keep a high chest, roll your shoulders back and down, and engage your core.

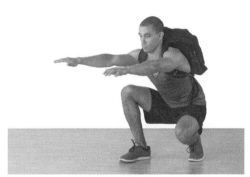

2–3: Without standing up from your squat, walk forward until your desired distance or time has been met.

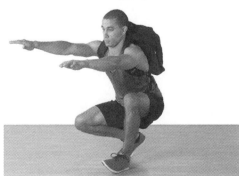

GORILLA WALK

TARGET: Shoulders, triceps, abs, quads

The gorilla walk allows you to easily switch between using your legs or arms as the dominant muscle group. Your whole body will tire out quickly, especially when using weights, which makes the gorilla walk a great conditioning movement.

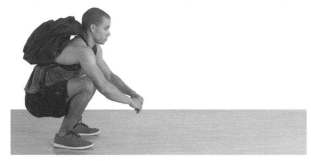

1: Place sandbags in a backpack and wear it on your back. Squat down until your hamstrings are resting on your calves. Keep a high chest, roll your shoulders back and down, and engage your core.]

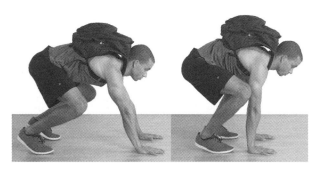

2–3: Put your hands down a foot in front of your feet and push yourself forward so that your feet land a foot in front of and in between your hands.

Continue this motion until your desired distance or time has been met.

INCHWORM WALK

TARGET: Abs, chest, shoulders, triceps, calves

The inchworm walk provides great work for the core and arms while also increasing hamstring mobility, something that people who spend a lot of time in an office chair or car can definitely use.

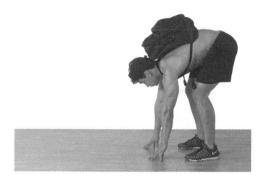

1: Place sandbags in a backpack and wear it on your back. Stand with your feet shoulder-width apart and your chest high, roll your shoulders back and down, and engage your core. Hinge at the hips and bring your hands to the ground. If your hamstrings keep your hands from reaching the ground, bend your knees as much as you need.

2–3: Walk your hands forward until your torso is completely parallel to the ground.

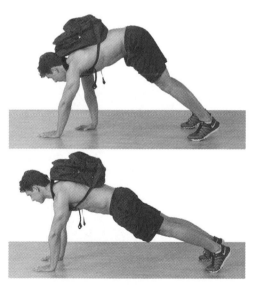

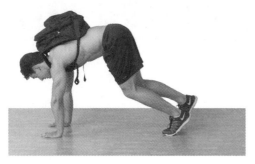

4–5: Then take small steps forward until your feet reach your hands.

Continue this motion until your desired distance or time is completed.

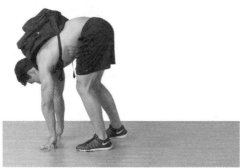

ARMY CRAWL

TARGET: Abs

The army crawl is a good movement for core stability, body control, and hip mobility.

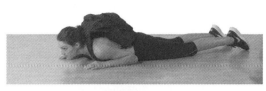

1: Place sandbags in a backpack and wear it on your back. Lie down on your stomach.

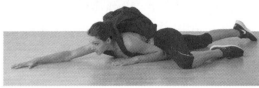

2: Crawl forward by reaching your right arm and left leg forward.

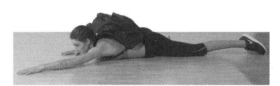

3: Repeat with the opposite limbs.

Continue this motion until your desired distance or time is completed.

SNATCH

TARGET: Glutes, hamstrings, quads shoulders

This very explosive movement is a great choice for athletes or anyone who wants to train like one. It's a tricky exercise made even more complex with the use of a sandbag, so really be sure to nail your form.

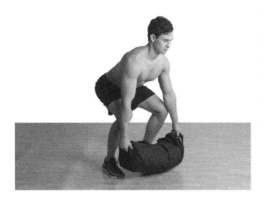

1: Stand with your feet shoulder-width apart and your chest high, roll your shoulders back and down, and engage your core. With the sandbag on the ground horizontally in front of you, hinge at the hips and bring your hands down to the handles or under the sandbag.

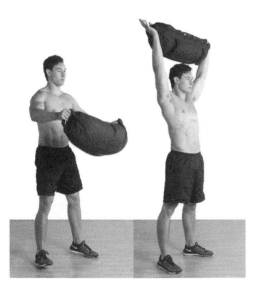

2–3: Use your glutes, hamstrings, and quads to explode upward, bringing the bag up above your head with arms almost completely extended.

CLEAN & JERK

TARGET: Glutes, hamstrings, quads, shoulders

Another Olympic weightlifting move, the clean and jerk also builds explosive strength. Using a sandbag rather than a barbell will force you to engage your core as much as possible, making the clean and jerk a true total-body killer.

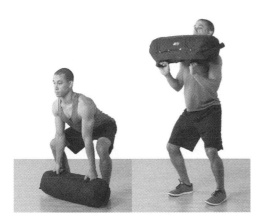

1–2: Stand with your feet shoulder-width apart and your chest high, roll your shoulders back and down, and engage your core. With the sandbag on the ground horizontally in front of you, hinge at the hips and bring your hands down to the handles or under the sandbag. Use your glutes, hamstrings, and quads to explode upward, bringing the bag up to your chest.

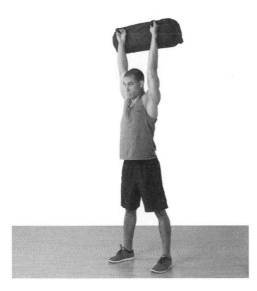

3: Adjust your grip, then use your legs and arms to drive the bag up over your head until your arms are almost completely extended.

THRUSTER

TARGET: Glutes, quads, shoulders

The thruster is one of the most demanding exercises in this book, making it great for those who like efficient workouts. It's also versatile enough to be used for conditioning if used with low weight, or strength training if used with heavy weight.

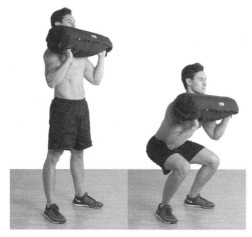

1–2: Stand with your feet shoulder-width apart and your chest high, roll your shoulders back and down, and engage your core. Hold the bag at chest level. Lower down into a squat.

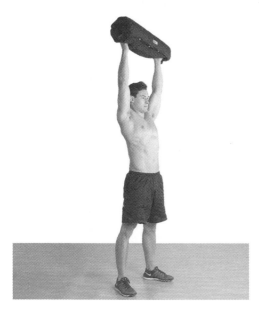

3: From the bottom of the squat, explode up with your legs and arms until the sandbag is over your head and your arms are almost completely extended.

THRUSTER WITH LUNGE

TARGET: Glutes, quads, shoulders

Want to make the thruster a bit more dynamic? Switch the squatting portion out for a lunge!

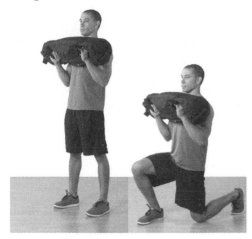

1–2: Stand with your feet shoulder-width apart and your chest high, roll your shoulders down and back, engage your core. Hold the sandbag at chest level. Step one leg forward to perform a lunge.

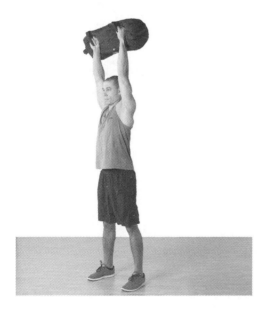

3: From the bottom of the lunge, explode up with your legs and arms until the sandbag is over your head and your arms are almost completely extended.

Repeat with the other leg.

OVERHEAD CHOP

TARGET: Glutes, hamstrings, shoulders, abs, triceps

This fun movement works both the front and back of the body. It's as good of an exercise as there is for standing core work.

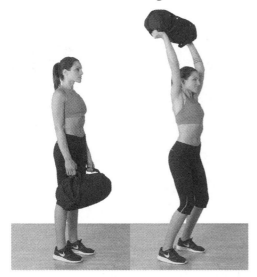

1–2: Stand with your feet shoulder-width apart and your chest high, roll your shoulders back and down, and engage your core. Start with the sandbag hanging in front of your legs. Explode upward with the legs, bringing the sandbag behind your head.

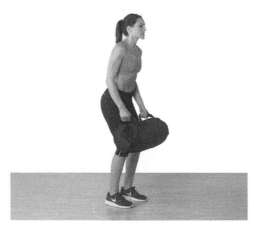

3: Without pause, use your core, shoulders, and arms to bring the bag back over your head and down to your knees to complete the rep.

SIDE CHOP

TARGET: Glutes, hamstrings, shoulders, abs

The side chop is a functional and effective core movement that also targets the glutes and hamstrings.

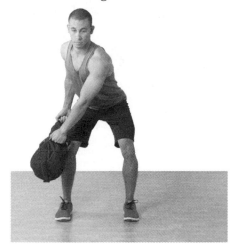

1: Stand with your feet shoulder-width apart and your chest high, roll your shoulders back and down, and engage your core. Start with the sandbag at your right knee.

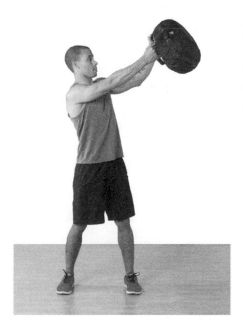

2: Use your whole body to bring it up to your left ear.

Smoothly lower the bag back down to knee level to complete the rep, and then perform the movement from the left knee to the right ear.

TURKISH GET-UP

TARGET: Glutes, quads, abs, shoulders

Although burpees get a lot of attention for being a full-body, cardiovascular challenge, Turkish get-ups take the challenge to another level. The form takes a bit to get down, but it's worth it. The get-up is an excellent addition to any workout, and is versatile enough to be used as a warm-up or finisher.

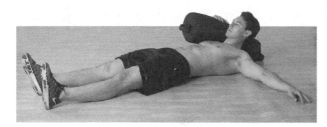

1: Lie on your back with the sandbag on your right shoulder.

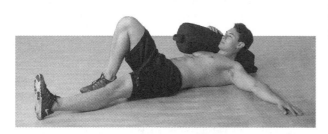

2: Bend your right knee and place your foot flat on the ground.

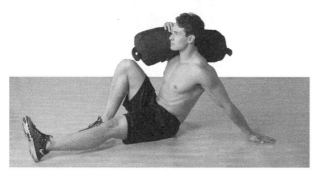

3: With your right foot still on the ground, use your core to sit up.

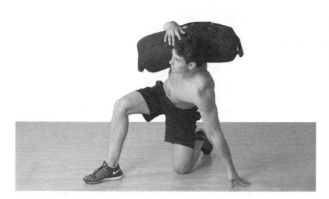

4: Use your left hand and right leg to swing your left leg back into a kneeling position.

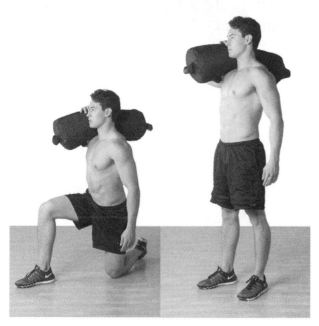

5–6: Use your left leg to lunge up into a standing position.

Reverse the motion to get back into the lying position to complete the rep.

SPRINT

TARGET: Glutes, hamstrings, quads

There's no greater cardiovascular challenge than an all-out uphill sprint with a sandbag. If you haven't ran full speed recently, take it slow at first. And don't skip a warm-up!

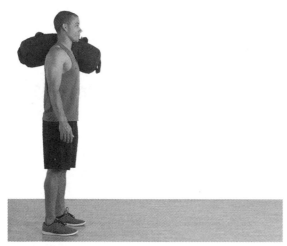

1: Stand with your chest high, roll your shoulders back and down, and engage your core. Hoist the sandbag onto one shoulder or carry it under your arm like a football.

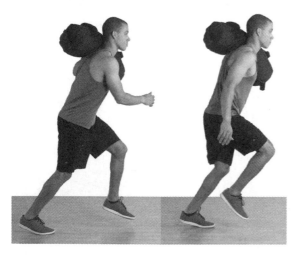

2–3: Sprint forward until your desired amount of time or distance is completed.

SIDE SHUFFLE SPRINT

TARGET: Glutes, quads

Rather than sticking to one-directional running, mix in some side shuffle sprints. Varying the motion can reduce wear and tear on the body, and keep engagement high.

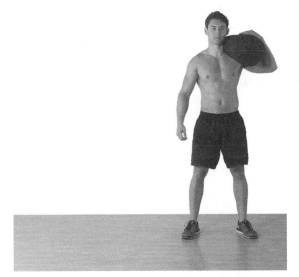

1: Stand with your chest high, roll your shoulders back and down, and engage your core. Hoist the sandbag onto one shoulder or carry it under your arm like a football.

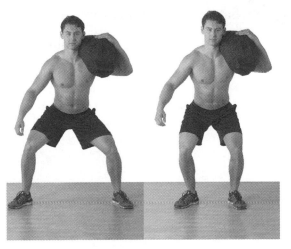

2–3: Keeping your knees bent throughout the movement, move your feet laterally in one direction until your desired amount of time or distance is completed, switching the sandbag to the other shoulder/arm after each interval.

CARIOCA SPRINT

TARGET: Glutes, quads

Carioca sprints are another fun twist to add to your conditioning regimen. A heavy sandbag makes the movement a good one for improving body control.

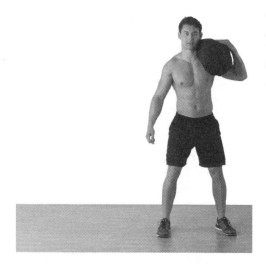

1: Stand with your chest high, roll your shoulders back and down, and engage your core. Hoist the sandbag onto one shoulder or carry it under your arm like a football.

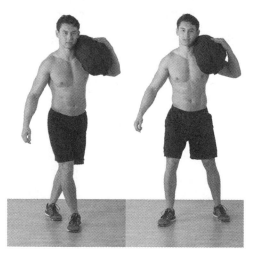

2–3: Shuffle to your right, with your left foot switching off between going in front or behind your right foot.

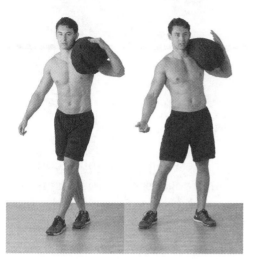

4–5: Shuffle to your left, with your right foot switching off between going in front or behind your left foot, switching the sandbag to the other shoulder/arm after each interval.

BACKPEDAL SPRINT

TARGET: Glutes, quads

To round out a sprint workout, be sure to include some backpedaling. It provides good work for the quads in addition to improving your ability to get back on defense.

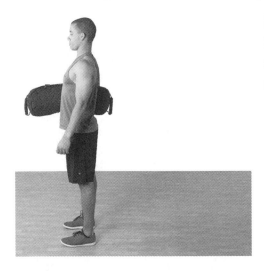

1: Stand with your chest high, roll your shoulders back and down, and engage your core. Hoist the sandbag onto one shoulder or carry it under your arm like a football.

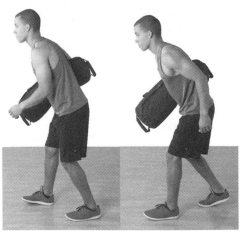

2–3: Sprint backward until your desired amount of time or distance has been completed, switching the sandbag to the other shoulder/arm after each interval.

SHOULDER FARMER'S WALK

TARGET: Glutes, quads

Farmer's walks are great for core stability and can also deliver a nice cardiovascular challenge if you hustle. Farmer's walks get truly dynamic by allowing you to move weight over distance.

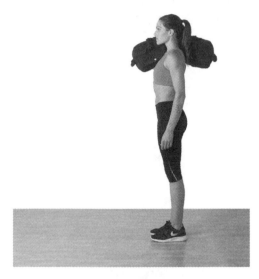

1: Stand with your chest high, roll your shoulders back and down, and engage your core. Hoist the sandbag up to one shoulder.

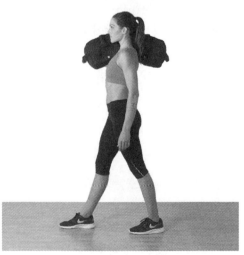

2: Walk until your desired amount of time or distance has been completed, switching the sandbag to the other shoulder after each interval.

SUITCASE FARMER'S WALK

TARGET: Glutes, quads

Suitcase farmer's walks allow you to strengthen your core in a different way while still working the legs. Be sure to keep the weight close to your body to reduce risk of injury.

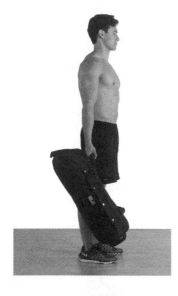

1: Stand with your chest high, roll your shoulders back and down, and engage your core. Hold the sandbag by the handles at your side.

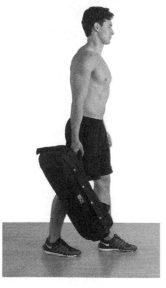

2: Walk until your desired amount of time or distance has been completed, switching the sandbag to the other hand after each interval.

OVERHEAD FARMER'S WALK

TARGET: Glutes, quads, shoulders

Overhead farmer's walks are absolutely brutal for the shoulders and arms while still giving the legs some work. Test your willpower and endurance by seeing how far you can go without lowering the weight.

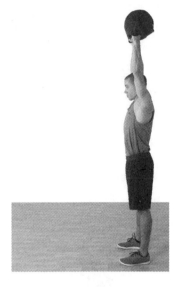

1: Stand with your chest high, roll your shoulders back and down, and engage your core. Hoist the sandbag overhead.

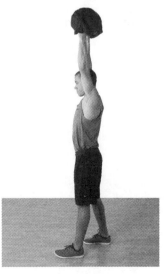

2: Walk until your desired amount of time or distance has been completed.

BURPEE

TARGET: Chest, quads, glutes, hamstrings

Burpees are both fun and devilishly tiring, which is perhaps why they're a favorite of boot camp instructors. They're versatile enough to start a workout, end a workout, or be a workout in and of themselves.

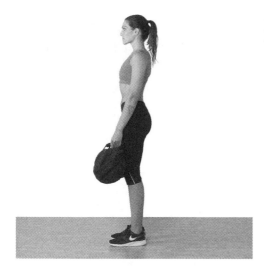

1: Stand with your chest high, roll your shoulders back and down, and engage your core. Hold the sandbag in front of your legs.

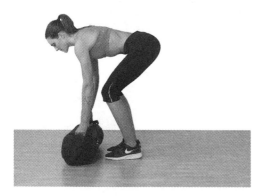

2: Hinge at the hips to place the sandbag down in front of you.

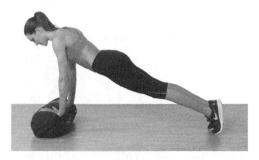

3: Place your hands on the sandbag and jump your feet back until you're in a plank position.

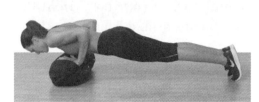

4: Do a push-up.

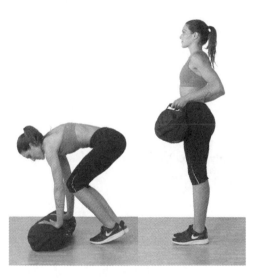

5–6: Pop up onto your feet and clean the sandbag up to your waist to complete the rep.

OVERHEAD PRESS VARIATION

To make the burpee even more intense, add an overhead press to the top of the movement. Use a heavy weight to intensely target the arms and shoulders; go lighter for an endurance challenge.

ROLLING BURPEE

TARGET: Glutes, quads, abs

To mix up the classic burpee, add a roll. Rolling burpees work best on soft surfaces, with green grass being my personal favorite.

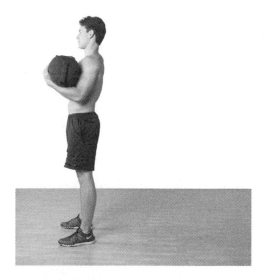

1: Stand with your chest high, roll your shoulders back and down, and engage your core. Hold the sandbag with your biceps or in a bear hug.

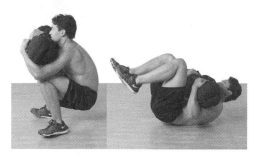

2–3: Drop down on onto your back.

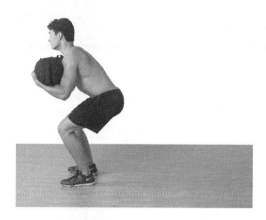

4: Rock backward and then forward until you can come up into the standing position.

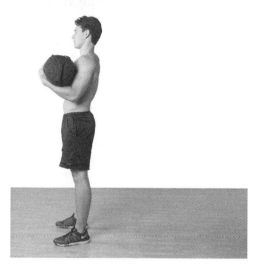

5: Clean the sandbag up to your waist to complete the rep.

SLED PULL

TARGET: Glutes, quads, calves

Sled pulls make you feel like a high-level athlete and are a great workout with heavy or light weight.

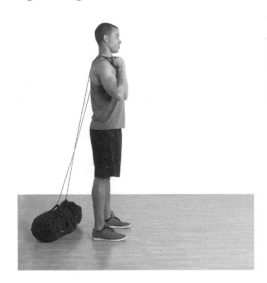

1: Stand with your chest high, roll your shoulders back and down, and engage your core. Loop a rope around the sandbag's handles or otherwise fasten the rope to the sandbag and hold the two rope ends in your hands.

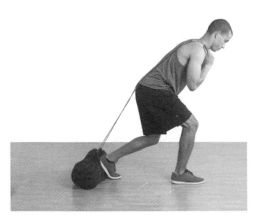

2: Pull the heavy sandbag until your desired distance or time has been completed.

You can either sprint for a more intense cardiovascular workout or lunge for a more strength-centric workout.

JUMPING JACK

TARGET: Calves

Jumping jacks aren't quite as easy as you remember from gym class when you add weight to the movement. It's a timeless calisthenic exercise nonetheless.

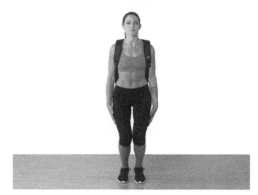

1: Place sandbags in a backpack and wear it on your back. Stand with your chest high, roll your shoulders back and down, and engage your core. Start with your hands at your sides and feet together.

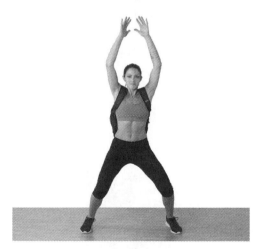

2: Jump your feet out so that they're now 24 inches apart while simultaneously swinging your hands overhead, also 24 inches apart.

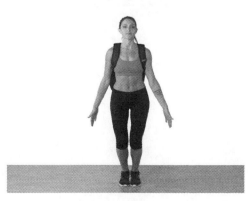

3: Jump back to starting position to complete the rep.

JUMPING ROPE

TARGET: Calves

Doing double-unders with resistance is a sure-fire way to feel like a heavyweight champ.

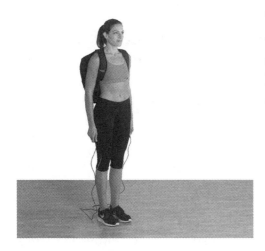

1: Place sandbags in a backpack and secure it tightly to your back, making sure it doesn't move around while you jump. Stand with your chest high, roll your shoulders back and down, and engage your core.

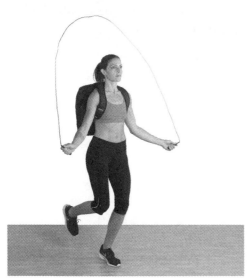

2: Jump while swinging the rope around your head until your desired amount of reps or time has been completed.

SANDBAG WHIP

TARGET: Shoulders, triceps

Sandbag whips are one of the few movements that test the endurance of the upper body. Be sure to use a light weight to reduce risk of injury.

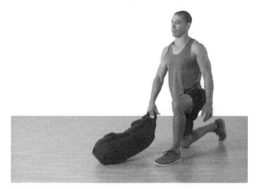

1: Sit or kneel on the ground with your chest high, roll your shoulders back and down, and engage your core. Grab the sandbag by one end.

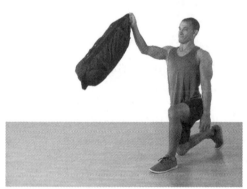

2: Lift it a few inches in the air.

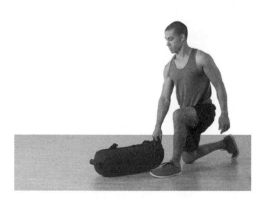

3: Slam it down against the ground.

Quickly repeat the motion without any pause. Continue until your desired amount of reps or time has been completed.

BOX JUMP

TARGET: Glutes, quads

Box jumps are a fun, playful way to explosively train the legs.

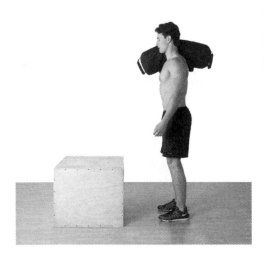

1: Stand with your chest high, roll your shoulders back and down, and engage your core. Hold the sandbag securely on one shoulder.

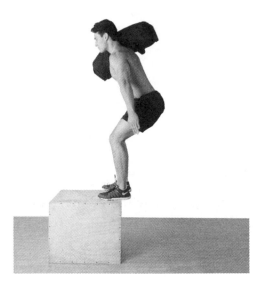

2: Explode off of two feet onto the 12- to 18-inch box in front of you.

Carefully step down from the box and then repeat the movement until your desired amount of reps or time has been completed.

ONE-LEG VARIATION

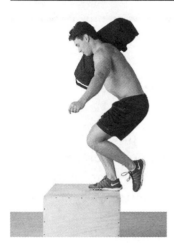

If normal box jumps feel too easy, try jumping off of one foot rather than two.

SPLIT LUNGE JUMP

TARGET: Glutes, quads

Few exercises can fatigue the legs as quickly as weighted split lunge jumps. They work very well as a finisher or when you need a super-quick workout.

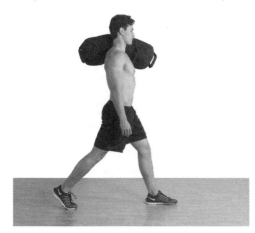

1: Stand with your chest high, roll your shoulders back and down, and engage your core. Place the sandbag on your shoulder and start with your right foot forward and your left foot back, about two feet apart.

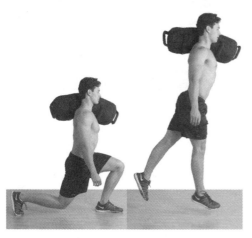

2–3: Lunge down until your left knee almost hits the ground and then explode up. While in the air, switch the places of your right and left feet.

Lunge down with your right leg and repeat the jump and foot switch. Switch the sandbag to the other shoulder after each set.

VERTICAL JUMP

TARGET: Glutes, quads

Practicing your vertical is a great way to improve your dunk. Like all max-effort exercises, be sure to properly warm up. The vertical jump can be performed off of one foot or two.

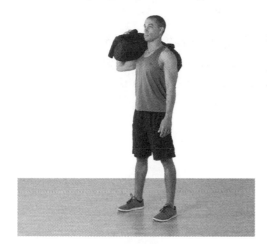

1: Hold a sandbag securely on one shoulder or wear a backpack filled with sandbags. Stand with your chest high, roll your shoulders back and down, and engage your core.

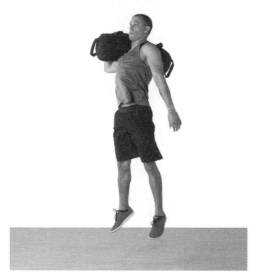

2: Jump as high as you can.

LONG JUMP

TARGET: Glutes, quads, hamstrings

The long jump can be performed by itself or done along with a long sprint, and can be done off of one foot or two. If you truly want to see how far you can go with soft wipeouts, head down to the beach and give it a go on sand.

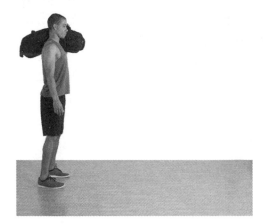

1: Hold a sandbag securely on one shoulder or wear a backpack filled with sandbags. Stand with your chest high, roll your shoulders back and down, and engage your core.

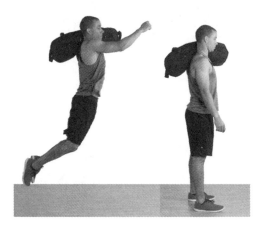

2–3: Jump as far forward as you can.

DISTANCE RUCK

TARGET: Glutes, quads, calves

The distance ruck is a true endurance challenge.

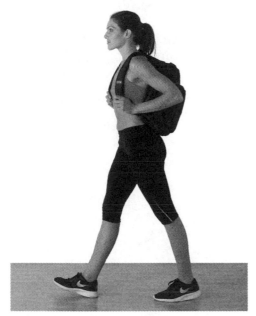

THE POSITION: Hoist a sandbag onto one shoulder or wear a backpack filled with sandbags. Stand with your chest high, roll your shoulders back and down, and engage your core. Walk until your desired distance is covered.

STAIR RUCK

TARGET: Glutes, quads

Add some lower-body intensity by walking up stairs or a steep hill. The stair ruck makes for an excellent combination of endurance and strength work.

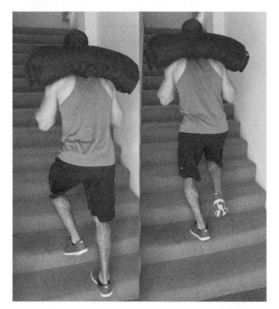

THE POSITION: Stand with your chest high, roll your shoulders back and down, and engage your core. Carry the sandbag on your shoulder, directly overhead, or in a bear hug. Walk up the stairs.

UPPER-BODY RUCK

TARGET: Glutes, quads, shoulders

Add some upper-body intensity to the ruck to make it a full-body endurance challenge. Go for a heavy weight to make the workout faster or use a lighter weight if you want a slow burn.

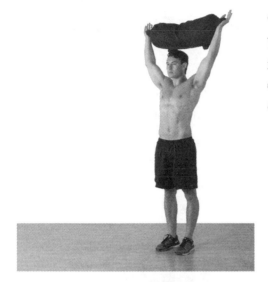

1: Stand with your chest high, roll your shoulders back and down, and engage your core. Walk forward while either holding a sandbag directly overhead, or switching it off between your right and left hands.

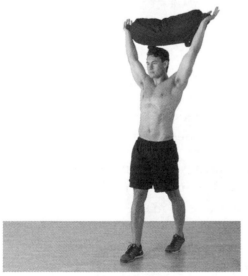

2: Continue walking until your desired amount of time has been reached.

WARMING UP

Here's a great collection of movements for warming up. Use the ones you like and toss the rest. Although it might seem like a pain, a quick warm-up is 100 times easier than sitting out a few months due to injury! All warm-up exercises should be done without a sandbag or any other added resistance.

JUMPING JACK

TARGET: Calves

Jumping jacks are an old-school calisthenic movement that can get the heart rate up in a hurry. They also get the upper body and arms loose, which are the parts of the body most often neglected during a warm-up.

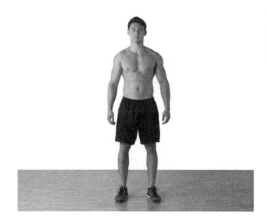

1: Stand with your chest high, roll your shoulders back and down, and engage your core. Start with hands at your sides.

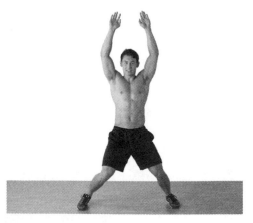

2: Jump your feet out so that they're now 24 inches apart while simultaneously swinging your hands overhead, also 24 inches apart.

Jump back to starting position to complete the rep. Continue the movement until your desired amount of time has been met.

MOUNTAIN CLIMBER

TARGET: Shoulders, chest, abs

A warm-up is most effective when it gets the heart rate up, and mountain climbers are a fantastic way to do that.

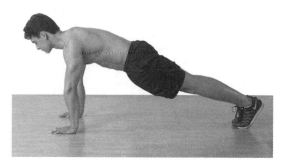

1: Place your hands on the floor, keeping your weight evenly distributed between your hands and feet.

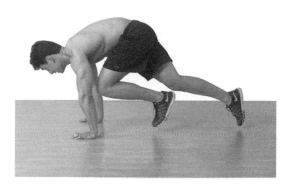

2: Jump your left foot forward 12 inches while simultaneously jumping your right foot back 12 inches.

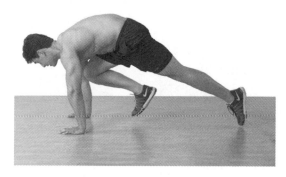

3: Jump your right foot forward 24 inches while simultaneously jumping your left foot back 24 inches.

Continue to switch the places of your right and left feet until your desired amount of reps or time has been met.

RUNNING IN PLACE

TARGET: Glutes, quads, calves

Running in place is a great warm-up move that can also help improve body control. One famous proponent of the exercise was the English runner Walter George, who claims it was an integral part of the training regimen that helped him become the fastest miler in the world in 1886 with a time of four minutes and twelve seconds.

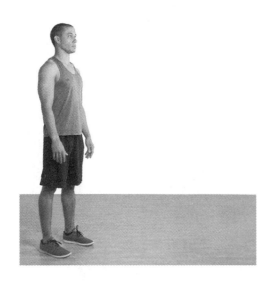

1: Stand with your chest high, roll your shoulders back and down, and engage your core.

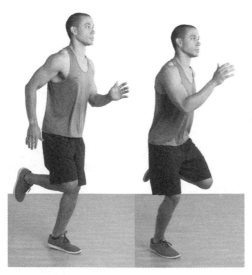

2–3: Pick up and put down your feet one at a time, aiming for them to be placed down in the same place over and over again at a rate of three steps per second.

Continue the movement until your desired amount of time has been met.

BUTT KICK

TARGET: Glutes, hamstrings, quads

Butt kicks help raise our body temperature and heart rate in addition to giving the quads a good warm-up. Don't worry if your heel doesn't actually reach your glutes; it's the thought that counts.

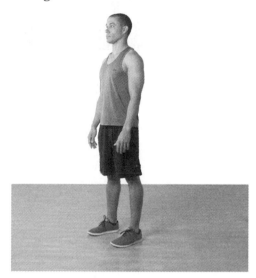

1: Stand with your chest high, roll your shoulders back and down, and engage your core.

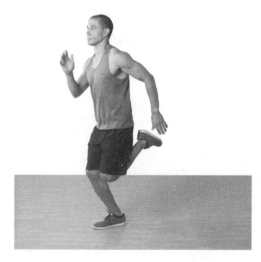

2: Jog forward for a few seconds and then change your running form so that your heels hit your glutes or at least get close on every step.

Continue the movement until your desired amount of time or distance has been met.

HIP GATE

TARGET: Hips

The hips are notoriously injury prone, especially as we age. The hip gate is a great warm-up movement that can increase comfort during the workout and decrease the chance of a tweak.

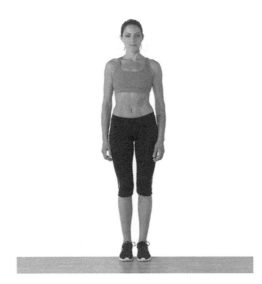

1: Stand with your chest high, roll your shoulders back and down, and engage your core.

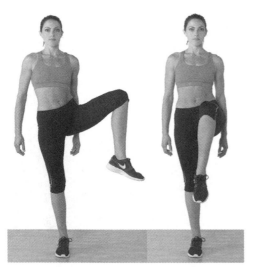

2–3: Walk forward and make a big outside-in half-circle with your left knee. Repeat with your right knee.

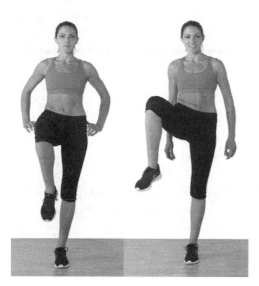

4–5: Walk forward and make a big inside-out half-circle with your right knee. Repeat with your left knee.

Continue to switch off between the inside-out half-circle and outside-in half-circle until your desired amount of time or distance has been met.

WINDMILL

TARGET: Shoulders

Windmills are a very helpful warm-up movement to perform if you're doing any upper-body exercises during your workout. It loosens up the shoulders, back, and pecs.

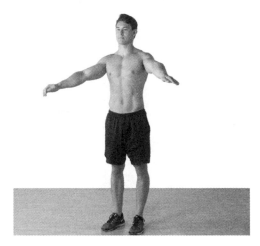

1–2: Stand with your chest high, roll your shoulders back and down, and engage your core. Make circles with your arms, first forward and then backward, until your desired amount of time or number of windmills have been completed. Use the biggest range of motion you can without feeling any discomfort.

Continue the movement until your desired amount of time or distance has been met.

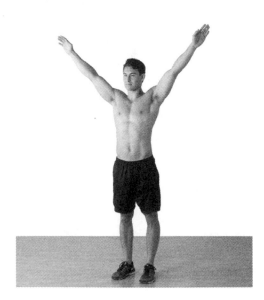

TOE KICK

TARGET: Hamstrings

Use this exercise in your warm-up if you have testy hamstrings. The key is to find your own stretching sweet spot with the exercise, being sure not to push it too far.

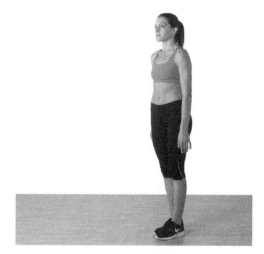

1: Stand with your chest high, roll your shoulders back and down, and engage your core.

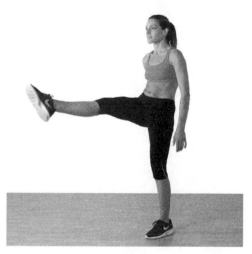

2: Kick your right foot up as high as it will comfortably go without forcing it.

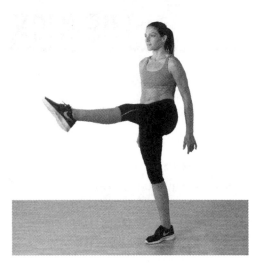

3: Repeat with your left foot, attempting to give the hamstrings a light stretch.

Continue the movement until your desired amount of time or distance has been met.

WALKING

TARGET: Glutes, quads, calves

Walking is a nice, gentle way to start any warm-up. The whole point of a warm-up is to start a workout off safely, and walking is the perfect conservative exercise.

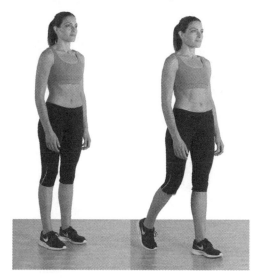

1–2: Stand with your chest high, roll your shoulders back and down, and engage your core. Put one foot in front of the other until your desired amount of time or distance has been met.

WORKOUT SHEET

MONDAY	
TUESDAY	
WEDNESDAY	
THURSDAY	
FRIDAY	
SATURDAY	
SUNDAY	

	WORKOUT SHEET
MONDAY	
TUESDAY	
WEDNESDAY	
THURSDAY	
FRIDAY	
SATURDAY	
SUNDAY	

INDEX

ACKNOWLEDGMENTS

Thanks to Mark Sisson for being the first person to introduce me to sandbag training through his website Marks Daily Apple, which has been a fantastic resource for me and many others over the years. Thanks to Vic Magary who renewed my interest in sandbag training with his article on Steve Kamb's website Nerd Fitness, which has also been a great resource for me and many others. Finally, thanks to all the folks at Ulysses Press for working with me, making me a better writer, and again giving me the privilege of seeing something I created for sale in stores.

ABOUT THE AUTHOR

Ben Hirshberg is a young author, health consultant, and entrepreneur from Seattle. He loves learning and applying anything that helps people live better, from nutrition to philosophy. He likes to cook, meditate, read, host parties, and go trail running. Download his manifesto for free at www.BenHirshberg.com.